The Psychosis and Mental Health Recovery Workbook

The **PSYCHOSIS** and **MENTAL HEALTH RECOVERY WORKBOOK**

Activities for Young Adults from ACT, DBT, and Recovery-Oriented CBT

Jennifer Gerlach

Foreword by Michelle Hammer

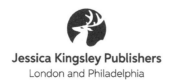

Jessica Kingsley Publishers
London and Philadelphia

First published in Great Britain in 2023 by Jessica Kingsley Publishers
An imprint of John Murray Press

1

Front cover image source: iStockphoto®.

Disclaimer: The information contained in this book is not intended to replace the
services of trained medical professionals or to be a substitute for medical advice.
You are advised to consult a doctor on any matters relating to your health, and in
particular on any matters that may require diagnosis or medical attention.

A CIP catalogue record for this title is available from the
British Library and the Library of Congress

ISBN 978 1 83997 732 9
eISBN 978 1 83997 733 6

Printed and bound in Great Britain by Bell & Bain Limited

Jessica Kingsley Publishers' policy is to use papers that are natural,
renewable and recyclable products and made from wood grown in
sustainable forests. The logging and manufacturing processes are expected
to conform to the environmental regulations of the country of origin.

Jessica Kingsley Publishers
Carmelite House
50 Victoria Embankment
London EC4Y 0DZ

www.jkp.com

John Murray Press
Part of Hodder & Stoughton Limited
An Hachette UK Company

To my sister

Foreword

As a mental health advocate who has traveled around the world telling my story of living with schizophrenia, I know that Jennifer Gerlach provides extremely helpful tools for mental health recovery in *The Psychosis and Mental Health Recovery Workbook*. She states in the book, "Mental health recovery means reclaiming what you have lost when you have been struggling with your mental health." When I read this quote, I thought of how many years I lost due to mismanaging my mental illness. I used to deny my mental illness, claim I didn't need my medication, and put myself in dangerous situations. Living with schizophrenia, I have struggled with paranoia, and it has hindered my ability to speak with therapists. A workbook like this, which I can keep in my possession, is exactly what I need.

This workbook brings a form of therapy straight to the reader. The questions it asks make the reader think deeply and reach previously unrealized insights about themselves. Each section starts with a personal story about the author before moving into the activity section. This gives the reader a look into the author's life and what living with mental illness is like for her.

The Psychosis and Mental Health Recovery Workbook should be given to all young adults who show signs of mental illness so that they, too, can benefit from the use of its wonderful tools. I hope that you, reader, will find this a useful resource in your recovery.

Michelle Hammer
Activist and Founder of Schizophrenic.NYC

Contents

Introduction

Dear Reader,

Each year, thousands of young adults struggle with mental health challenges such as bipolar disorder, major depression, and psychosis. As many as one in five people will face such a challenge in their lifetime. If you are reading this book, you or someone you love might be part of that one-in-five statistic. I am too.

Years ago, at age 13, I experienced a psychiatric hospitalization followed by several months of me trying to prove to everyone around me that I was not "crazy" and that I did not need all of the help being offered to me. I did not want to think of myself as the caricature that I had drawn in my mind of what it means to have a mental illness. The truth is, I was not crazy and neither are you.

Experiences like hearing voices, paranoia, depression, and mania are normal reactions to a variety of circumstances and health conditions. Having a mental health condition or any of the above experiences does not mean that you are "crazy" or that you have to give up on your hopes and dreams. Support from friends, family, and treatment providers can help you on your way.

The skills reviewed in this book draw from psychotherapies including Recovery-Oriented Cognitive Therapy (CT-R) (Beck *et al.* 2020), Dialectical Behavioral Therapy (DBT) (Linehan 2014), and Acceptance Commitment Therapy (ACT) (Luoma, Hayes and Walser 2007), which are considered evidence-based treatments for psychosis and related conditions. In other words, a bunch of scientists and mental health folks have done studies that show that these particular therapies work in moving people away from getting stuck in unwanted experiences and toward their goals.

As you move through this book, feel free to skip ahead and dip in and out as you find topics of interest to you. You may also choose to work through this book with a therapist or family member for extra support.

Still, this workbook is no replacement for your own therapy or psychiatric intervention. If you find yourself affected by the symptoms discussed in this book, I strongly encourage you to engage with a mental health professional whom you can trust. They can work together with you to create a recovery plan.

Recovery from psychosis and other mental health conditions is absolutely possible. It is common to have bumps along the way. If at any point you feel like giving up on your journey, please know that help is available and tell someone right away. You can find contact details for helplines that are available 24 hours a day, seven days a week in the back of this book.

Jen

Part 1

MORE THAN A DIAGNOSIS

1

What Is Mental Health Recovery?

At 13, I did not know what a mental illness was. That was before my hospitalization. After my hospitalization, I had, on one hand, a diagnosis I did not understand and, on the other hand, all this shame and embarrassment. How would I explain the two weeks of school I missed to everyone? What about how I was acting before? My psychiatric hospitalization marked the beginning of a long road of multiple diagnoses, treatments, strategies, and hard work toward my recovery. I have defined my recovery as living the best life I can toward what is important to me, even with my mental health condition. The day after my hospitalization, I don't think I would have thought that could even be possible.

Recovery is a word meaning to get back something you have lost. You may have overheard fellow customers at a coffee shop talking about a country's economic "recovery," or you may know someone in "recovery" from a substance abuse disorder. Mental health recovery means reclaiming what you have lost when you have been struggling with your mental health and moving toward your values.

Each person gets to author their recovery. Everyone's healing is different. For most, recovery involves some re-engaging with life, be it restoring friendships, re-entering school, or re-focusing on goals. It could also mean getting a handle on mental health symptoms that are preventing you from living your best life. Still, you do not have to be "symptom-free" to be in recovery. It is more about adapting so that you can move toward the good things than it is about making all the bad things go away.

If you were recently diagnosed with a mental health condition or had a mental health crisis, you may be struggling to imagine a situation different from the one you are in now. Please have hope. Millions of people have recovered from mental health conditions, including psychosis, and you can too. No one can tell you what your recovery should look like; that is up to you. There are no "wrong" answers. Your vision for your recovery might (and likely will) change over time as you move forward. This is normal and good. Take some time on the following page to reflect on what you wish for your recovery.

What Are Your Hopes for Your Recovery?

Check off your hopes for your recovery.

- ☐ Better understanding my experience
- ☐ Reconnecting with friends
- ☐ Relief from mental health symptoms
- ☐ Feeling happier
- ☐ Recovering my credibility and respect from others
- ☐ Rebuilding my self-respect
- ☐ Preparing for career and education goals
- ☐ Having things in my life again aside from mental health treatment
- ☐ Accepting my experience
- ☐ Recovering from the trauma of my experience
- ☐ Feeling a greater sense of meaning
- ☐ Feeling a greater sense of achievement

What other hopes do you have for your recovery?

_____

_____

_____

_____

_____

_____

_____

Understanding Your Experiences

When I first received help, I did not understand my experiences. Everything felt so out of control. I didn't know if anyone could understand. Having words for my challenges was helpful, but those words also felt intimidating. One of the first diagnoses I was given was "psychosis." That word made me think of the word "psycho"—reminiscent of horror films and things I wanted nothing to do with. My diagnosis changed over and over. I felt like I could no longer just be me but was at the mercy of whatever label that was currently stamped on my chart. But learning about my challenges and especially meeting others who had "been there" helped a lot. Going to a support group and a mental health recovery class gave me a sense that I am not alone.

Mental health challenges include a variety of difficulties involving our emotions and thoughts. Dealing with mental health challenges such as depression, paranoia, and hearing voices can be scary and interrupt our daily lives. Still, as many as one in five adolescents will deal with a mental health condition at some point in their life (Kieling *et al.* 2011). Chances are that you know several people in your daily life who are coping with such difficulties as these.

Psychosis is a specific kind of mental health challenge that can cause symptoms such as:

- voices
- seeing things other people can't
- unusual beliefs (such as that you are receiving secret messages or could be the target of a conspiracy)
- paranoia
- very scattered thoughts
- changes in behavior
- trouble with motivation
- difficulty concentrating
- feeling less social
- not wanting to do things you used to enjoy
- feeling very restless
- difficulty putting words or sentences together.

Not all people who experience one or more of these symptoms have a mental health condition. Symptoms like these can also be caused by experiences and conditions such as substance use, extreme stress, physical health conditions, and sleep deprivation. Psychosis and other mental health conditions can only be diagnosed by a mental health professional.

Having a psychotic disorder or other mental health condition does not mean someone is "crazy." In fact, under enough physical or emotional stress, anyone will experience some mental health challenges. The behaviors a person might engage in while experiencing a mental health condition may be confusing to those around them but make sense given what the person living with the condition is experiencing.

In Japan, psychosis is called an "integration disorder" (Sato 2006) because it is a health condition that affects how we integrate sensory and emotional information and thoughts. For some people, psychosis can be temporary. For others, psychosis can last longer. Someone can also have an initial psychotic episode and then have a second psychotic break some time after. Understanding your particular pattern of challenges can help you take steps toward your recovery.

Research suggests that most people who have a mental health episode will recover (Slade & Longden 2015). Learning from others with mental health challenges and reaching out to good information can be an excellent first step in regaining a sense of wellbeing and meaning.

Your Experiences

Listed below are common mental health challenges. Check the boxes of symptoms that you have experienced.

☐ Hearing voices
☐ Feeling like someone might be out to get you
☐ A vague feeling that you could be in danger
☐ Feeling very down
☐ Having trouble keeping track of your thoughts
☐ Feeling like you may have special powers such as reading minds
☐ Feeling like you could be sending or receiving telepathic messages
☐ A belief that you have been sent on a special or top-secret mission
☐ Feeling restless
☐ Talking more than usual
☐ Depression
☐ Anxiety
☐ Talking less than usual
☐ Seeing things other people cannot see
☐ Feeling things when there is nothing there (such as bugs on your skin)
☐ Having difficulties putting words together
☐ Being less interested in things you used to enjoy
☐ Trouble concentrating
☐ Trouble relaxing
☐ Feeling very high or unstoppable
☐ Having too many thoughts at once (this is also called racing thoughts)
☐ _____
☐ _____

Which three challenges are most getting in the way of your life right now?

1. _____
2. _____
3. _____

What goals do you hope to return to as you work through these challenges?

1. _____
2. _____
3. _____

Reflect on this: What will be the best part about moving toward your recovery?

_____

_____

_____

_____

_____

_____

_____

_____

_____

_____

3

You Are More Than a Diagnosis

Before going to the hospital, I saw myself as a student, a dog lover, and a probably overly enthusiastic school band member. The months after my hospitalization felt like a blur where the only role I played in life was "patient." I used to be someone to have a quirky sense of humor and some eccentricities. After receiving a list of diagnoses, the lens I use to view myself changed. Was I "sad" or depressed? Was I "happy" or manic? I even questioned whether I could trust my judgment or perceptions anymore.

Still, in time, I remembered that I am still me. My emotions are real. My experiences are valid. I am more than a diagnosis.

Experiencing a mental health crisis can mark a transition in someone's life. It is important to know this: You are the same person that you were before you knew you had a mental health condition. The eyes you were born with are the same eyes reading this page, and you are the person behind those eyes.

In Acceptance Commitment Therapy (ACT), this is called the observing self. You can think of the observing self as that you behind your eyes. Not the thoughts, emotions, or perceptions that that you is experiencing but you.

TRY THIS

Sing a tone. Listen to the tone. Are you the tone? Are you the voice? Are you your ears? The observing self is the you hearing the sound—the you watching you do these things.

Mental health symptoms can affect your thoughts and emotions. Regardless of whether or not you have a mental health condition, the person behind your eyes is still the same. You are not your thoughts or emotions; you are more than these. There is much more to a person than an illness.

If you have recently had a mental health crisis, you are probably hearing words like "patient" and "diagnosis" more often. It might be silly to say, but please remember you are more than that. At your core, you are not a patient or client. You are not a diagnosis. You are a person. Remember and appreciate the parts of you beyond your illness.

Your Strengths

Create an image that represents you. Think about your strengths, your supports, and your passions. This can be a self-portrait, an animal with qualities you relate to, or something totally different. Think about the person you are beyond your illness.

Your Roles

What roles are important to you?

Check off roles here that are part of your life:

- ☐ Being a sibling
- ☐ Being a student
- ☐ Being a son, daughter, or child
- ☐ Being a member of a certain club or group
- ☐ Being an advocate
- ☐ Being a partner
- ☐ Being a friend
- ☐ Being a part of your faith or other spiritual practice

☐ _____

☐ _____

Of these roles, which three are most important to you right now?

1. _____

2. _____

3. _____

Remember, you are also more than any of these roles. Think a second about what it is like to be the person behind your eyes. What does the world look like from your perspective? How are you engaging your "observing self" (the self that is here, right now, reading this sentence)?

4

Your Strengths and Values

For a time, I forgot what I was good at. My life had been all about music and band before the hospital. After, concentrating or having motivation to play my instrument proved difficult. I thought I was smart, but my grades dropped quite a bit with my mental health. Something that I didn't lose, though, was curiosity. I value carving new paths and exploring. This helped me through as I caught up and found my way.

Strengths are your positive qualities. You can have strengths in things you know, things you can do, cultural strengths, strengths that come from life experience, character strengths, and more.

Values are the assets we strive for. Moving toward a value is like moving in a direction on a compass; there is always more to be done. For example, each day you can take a step toward being kind, but no matter how hard you try, a sign will never drop from the skies that says, "Welcome to kind!" It's not a destination you arrive at, but something you inch toward throughout your life. You don't have to wait to achieve your value with some grand action.

Accessing your strengths and values is something you can practice every day. If you have difficulties identifying strengths, it may be helpful to ask someone you trust what they see as your strengths or to make a point to listen when you receive positive feedback. You can also pay attention to when you feel a sense of meaning, accomplishment, and positive emotions. Those times represent a sparkle that will point you in the direction of your values.

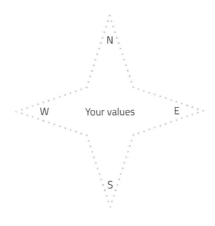

Your Values

Check out this list of values and feel free to add your own.

- ☐ Compassion
- ☐ Love
- ☐ Curiosity
- ☐ Honesty
- ☐ Resilience
- ☐ Hope
- ☐ Critical thinking
- ☐ Kindness
- ☐ Faith
- ☐ Never giving up
- ☐ Staying active
- ☐ Strength
- ☐ Security
- ☐ Trust

- ☐ Self-respect
- ☐ Self-compassion
- ☐ Self-love
- ☐ New ideas
- ☐ Forgiveness
- ☐ Doing my best
- ☐ Generosity
- ☐ Trust
- ☐ Connection
- ☐ Trying new things
- ☐ _____
- ☐ _____
- ☐ _____

Which of these values are most important for you...

As a friend?

1. _____
2. _____
3. _____

In your work and/or schooling?

1. _____
2. _____
3. _____

As a member of your family?

1. _____
2. _____
3. _____

As a human being or member of your community?

1. _____

2. _____

3. _____

Close your eyes and take a moment to think about a time when you were at your best. Maybe you were singing in a choir concert, or enjoying a milkshake with friends. Think about the qualities and values that were drawn out for you at that moment. Savor this experience. Create a mental experience of what you see, what you hear, and most of all what it feels like to be in this space. When you are ready, open your eyes and create an image that reflects your vision.

Your Inspiration Playlist

As I got treatment for my mental health challenges, I often encountered others who were struggling. In a sense, I felt that I was not alone, but I often wondered, "Does anyone make it through this?" One day, I saw a flyer at the local library advertising a mental health recovery class at a local church. I attended. There I met two people living good lives with a mental health diagnosis. That gave me hope. I later learned that many people I admire live with or could have qualified for a mental health diagnosis. Great people like Demi Lovato and Abraham Lincoln have struggled with their mental health. Not only is it possible to make it through this, but you can also thrive with a mental health diagnosis.

When preparing for your recovery journey, gathering resources for support and inspiration is essential. Hearing from others in recovery from a mental health challenge can be an excellent source of strength. Many people also find certain songs inspirational or energizing in their lyrics, rhythms, and melody. You can use music strategically to lift your spirits and drive forward in your recovery.

Of course, music is not the only means of available inspiration. You might find inspiration in hearing stories from others about how they overcame adversity and achieved their goals. Or you might find inspiration in thinking about how far you have come.

You can find inspiration in mantras, quotes, films, views of nature, art, or celebration of your faith. You might try a few different things as you learn what inspires you. If you feel uninspired at first, keep searching. Inspiration can take time to find.

Your Soundtrack

What songs or other media give you energy or inspiration when you need it?

1. _____

2. _____

3. _____

If there were a song for your journey and strength, a "fight song" of sorts, what would it be called?

_____

You can consider this "fight song" as a kind of mantra or cheer to remind you of your strength. Another way to remember could be through creating a symbol.

Draw a symbol for your strength.

Part 2

TAMING STRESS

6

When Genetics Meet Overwhelming Stress

When I first started struggling with mental health symptoms, I went through several neurological tests. My providers were trying to rule out any physical causes for my problems. Ironically, this gave me hope. I thought if they found something physical going on with me, it would mean that this wasn't my fault.

I thought that having a mental illness meant that my providers believed my difficulties were "all in my head," and that I could make those go away at will. I knew that I couldn't make it stop. I tried. Having something out of my control like that scared me. Sometimes I wondered if these labels just meant I am a bad person. What I didn't know is that mental health conditions likely have a physical basis too, which can be set off by environmental triggers such as stress. My condition was not something I asked for or something I could make go away at will.

While the exact cause of most mental health challenges is unknown, one hypothesis is the diathesis-stress model. According to this idea, the origin usually lies in an interaction between biological vulnerability and stress. It is no one's fault and it is not a character flaw (Pruessner *et al.* 2016).

The diathesis-stress model suggests that when anyone is under enough stress, they will be at risk of mental health symptoms. Biological vulnerabilities linked up with genetics can also impact whether a person develops a mental health condition. For example, a person with a biological parent or sibling with a mental illness is at a much greater risk of having a mental illness even if they do not know that family member (Ingraham & Kety 2000).

You can think of it like this—we all have a certain level of stress which could put us at risk for having mental health symptoms. Genetics and other influences determine each of our natural abilities to resist the impact of stress. It does not mean you are "crazy" or will never get through this.

Having a sensitivity to stress also does not mean that you cannot handle stress at all. Within the following chapters, we will explore several ways to increase your resilience to stress. Many people living with mental health conditions live good lives and adapt new ways to surf through stress effectively.

Common Myths

Have you heard any of these common myths about mental health challenges?

☐ If I was a stronger person, I would not have gotten a mental illness
☐ Someone has to be to blame if someone has a mental health condition
☐ Psychosis is another word for crazy
☐ People with mental health conditions are weak and can't deal with life
☐ Mental health conditions are not "real" medical illnesses

How can you remind yourself that these things are not true when/if these thoughts come up?

_____

_____

_____

_____

_____

_____

_____

_____

Remember a time when you dealt with a stressful event particularly well. What did you do that allowed you to cope so well?

_____

_____

_____

_____

_____

_____

_____

_____

What Stresses You Out?

Avoiding stress felt non-negotiable at the beginning of my recovery. I worried that if I pushed myself too much, I might get ill again. Here is something I have learned—sometimes avoiding stress adds stress. Things like playing music, staying as on top of school as I could, and moving forward with life mattered. Not doing those things was just as, if not more, stressful than doing them. I did not have to push myself past my limits, but I didn't have to give up either. Everyone has limits, and sometimes I do need to decrease stress. But I don't have to steer clear of all stress. What stresses one person out might not bother another person. Taking into account what stresses you out can help you plan to block unnecessary stress and cope with it when necessary.

Stress is a little different for everyone. We all have stress triggers, but not everyone's triggers are the same. Different things stress different people out to different degrees. For example, some people find social gatherings stressful. Others find social gatherings a source of stress relief.

Knowing your triggers and the extent to which these affect you is an empowering way of coping. Just because something adds stress to your life does not mean you have to cut it out of your life, but it can be useful to know. Knowing you have a day ahead which contains several stressors could be a good signal to ramp up your use of stress shields. It might also be helpful to spread out high-stress activities over several days so that you do not get overwhelmed with too much stress at one time.

Listening to your body is another way to get a sense of when you are stressed and can help you identify the sources of it. Sometimes we feel stress in our bodies before we feel it emotionally. If you notice your muscles tensing or your heart racing, ask yourself, "Is something causing me stress?" If you notice these things, know this may be your body's way of gearing up to tackle a challenge.

Common Stressors

Mark how stressful you find each common stressor below by shading in the triangle to the level of stress each listed item causes you.

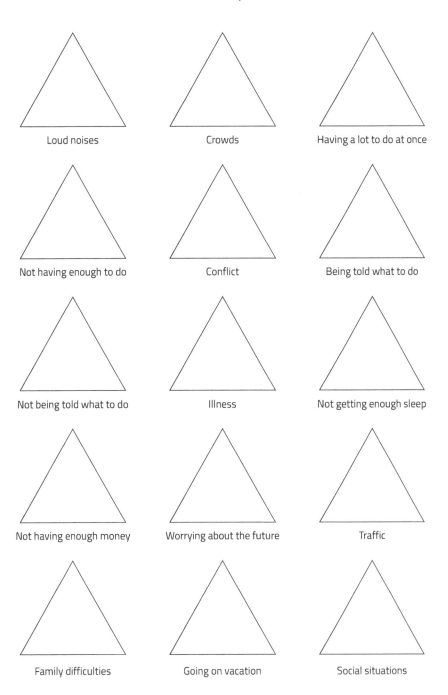

Loud noises	Crowds	Having a lot to do at once
Not having enough to do	Conflict	Being told what to do
Not being told what to do	Illness	Not getting enough sleep
Not having enough money	Worrying about the future	Traffic
Family difficulties	Going on vacation	Social situations

Stress Shields

I used to avoid stressful situations. Here is the problem: There are so many good things in life that cause stress. What I do now is do things each day that serve as shields between me and life stress. I keep close track of my sleep and try my best to get enough sleep each night. I make sure I talk to someone important to me every day. I journal. These strategies help me guard against stress.

If you were going into a battle, would you want to have a sword, a shield, or both? Stress shields are the things we do to protect ourselves from stress even before that stress comes up. Stress shields can help us to cope ahead of time with stress by strengthening our reserves to deal with stress before the storm hits.

Chances are that you already are using some stress shields every day— things like listening to music, spending time in nature, or using a planner to keep your schedule from getting too overwhelmed. Carrying with you one or more stress shields builds up your strength for times when stress is harder to handle. You may already be using many good stress shields *and* there are likely more shields that you can add to your arsenal. Check out the activity that follows to take inventory of your stress shields.

Stress Shields

These are stress shields.

Shade in shields you already use.
Circle shields you would be willing to try.

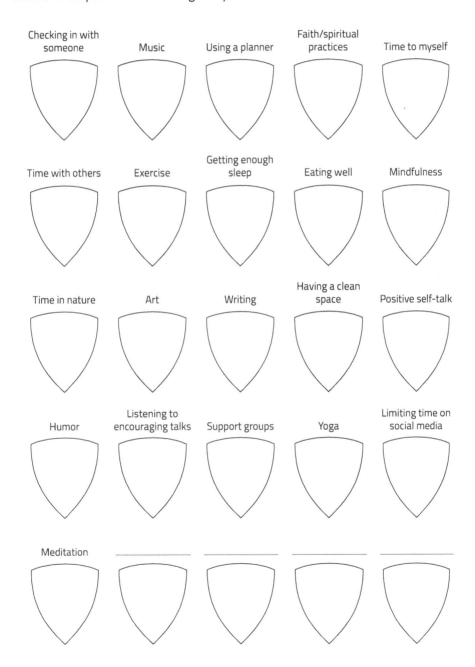

Checking in with someone   Music   Using a planner   Faith/spiritual practices   Time to myself

Time with others   Exercise   Getting enough sleep   Eating well   Mindfulness

Time in nature   Art   Writing   Having a clean space   Positive self-talk

Humor   Listening to encouraging talks   Support groups   Yoga   Limiting time on social media

Meditation

Warning Signs of Stress

I have learned that the earlier I can identify when I am stressed, the better I can cope with my stress. Sometimes my body knows that I am stressed before I do. Trouble sleeping at night or headaches are both signs to me that stress has entered the room. Once I notice that I am feeling stressed, I can take action. Sometimes this is as simple as taking a walk outside and listening to the birds. Other times, this might mean switching up my activities for the day so that I do not have so much piled on at once. At times, I take the sign that I am feeling stressed and carry on. Noticing my stress before it reaches a critical level has been key to maintaining my wellness.

Stress is something that we all experience throughout life. Our minds and bodies use stress to alert us to potential danger and gear us up to protect ourselves. In the right situations, stress can give us the motivation and energy we need to handle what we need to handle.

Still, when out of control, stress can trigger mental health difficulties. It is normal to have trouble concentrating or to feel irritable or anxious when stressed. For some, stress can also trigger more significant problems such as hearing voices, panic attacks, or paranoia. When stress is overwhelming, it can interfere with doing things you need to do.

Recognizing your early warning signs of stress will help you notice when your stress level is getting higher while you still have time to tackle it. The earlier you catch your stress, the more time you have to create a strategy to deal with stress at the moment to prevent damage.

TRY THIS

Focus on your body, beginning at the bottom of your toes and moving slowly up through your legs, your trunk, your stomach, your chest, your neck, your face, and your neck. Notice any tension you feel in each of these areas. If it feels right to stretch, stretch. Often we carry stress in our body without even knowing it. This exercise is called a body scan. Body scans can help you to build up awareness of stress in your body and help you to notice stress earlier so that you can work through it.

Your Signs of Stress

Shade or color the common signs of stress that you relate to.

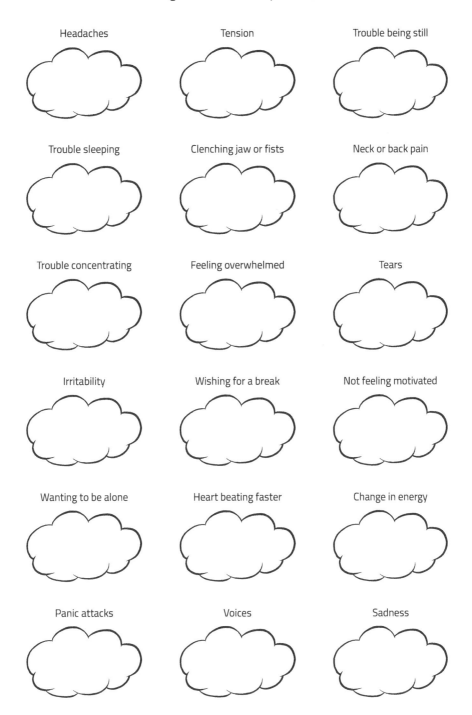

Headaches

Tension

Trouble being still

Trouble sleeping

Clenching jaw or fists

Neck or back pain

Trouble concentrating

Feeling overwhelmed

Tears

Irritability

Wishing for a break

Not feeling motivated

Wanting to be alone

Heart beating faster

Change in energy

Panic attacks

Voices

Sadness

10

Coping With Stress

After going to the hospital, people kept talking to me about "coping" with stress. At first, I thought this meant avoiding anything I thought could stress me out. Family gatherings made me nervous, so I wouldn't go. Learning to drive caused me anxiety, so I skipped the class. I wanted to do these things, but stress scared me. As my world got smaller, I thought there had to be a better way. I found a middle ground. I wrote down everything that stressed me out at the time and split it into what I can and cannot avoid. But that was just the first step. I learned that some things are worth the stress. Things like time with my grandmother and driving. I can take steps ahead of time, in the moment, and after to protect my mental health. Stress is not the boss of me.

Knowing that stress is a trigger for mental health problems, you may worry that you must avoid stress as much as possible and give up on anything stressful. While decreasing stress in the short term may be helpful to your mental health, the truth is we cannot get rid of all stress. A lot of central things in life like relationships, school, work, and recreation are full of stress.

Rather than avoiding stress altogether, it is more workable to create a strategy for coping with the stress that comes our way. This way, we can still enjoy the good without becoming overwhelmed by the stress that often follows. As you get to know better your needs in stressful situations, build up shields to protect from the impacts of stress pre-emptively, and create strategies for coping with stress in the moment, you will gain a stronger sense of resilience in the face of this trigger.

As your stressors and stress levels change, the assortment of skills you use will change too. With a strong arsenal of strategies, you can cope and do what you enjoy.

Coping With Stress Plan

Think about some of the stresses in your life.

What stressors in your life are unavoidable?

1. _____
2. _____
3. _____

What strategies could you use to cope with each of these unavoidable stressors?

- ☐ Check in with a supportive friend or mentor
- ☐ Schedule time alone
- ☐ Make sure to get enough sleep
- ☐ Make sure I have good food to eat
- ☐ Positive self-talk
- ☐ Remember why this stress is worth it
- ☐ Practice deep breathing
- ☐ Practice mindfulness

- ☐ _____
- ☐ _____

What stressors in your life are avoidable?

1. _____
2. _____
3. _____

What is the cost of avoiding each of these? (e.g., missing out on time with friends)

1. _____
2. _____
3. _____

What avoidable stressors in your life are worth moving toward?

1. _____
2. _____
3. _____

What strategies could you use to cope with each of these avoidable stressors?

- ☐ Check in with a supportive friend or mentor
- ☐ Schedule time alone
- ☐ Make sure to get enough sleep
- ☐ Make sure I have good food to eat
- ☐ Positive self-talk
- ☐ Remember why this stress is worth it
- ☐ Practice deep breathing
- ☐ Practice mindfulness

☐ _____

☐ _____

Part 3

DEALING WITH VOICES, PARANOIA, AND NEGATIVE SYMPTOMS

11

You Are Stronger Than Voices

There was a time when I had loud, voice-like thoughts in my mind on most days. These thoughts felt separate from my own, which made the experience quite upsetting. I named the thoughts "the voice." The voice would tell me all the bad things about myself, that no one liked me, and worse. It took time for me to recognize that the voice had no real power and to give myself the kindness I needed during this experience.

Hearing voices is a common experience; however, it is often misunderstood. Know that you are stronger than your voices. If voices ever tell you to do something, tell a trusted adult, such as a mental health professional, as soon as possible. Voices cannot physically harm you and you do not have to do anything that the voices say. Hearing voices does not make you "crazy," and it is nothing to be ashamed of.

Voices can happen inside your head or outside your head. Some people hear voices that talk to them, while others hear more than one voice talking to each other. Voices are often negative, telling you bad things about yourself or that you should not trust others. Some people hear positive voices. Sometimes making out what a voice is saying is difficult. Other times voices can be so loud that it can be hard to separate your own thoughts from the voice. Mental health treatment can help to minimize the intrusiveness of this painful symptom.

If you hear voices outside your head, there may be times when it is difficult to tell what is a person talking in real life and what is the voice of your mind. In group settings, this can be especially hard. One trick you can try is to watch the lips of a person talking. If you do not see their lips moving, you may be hearing a voice rather than the person. Another strategy is asking the person you are talking with to repeat what they said to verify that you heard them correctly. People mishear each other all the time, and so you can do this without revealing that you are having trouble with voices if you do not want to.

TRY THIS

Mindfulness for coping with voices

While hearing voices can interfere with practicing certain mindfulness activities, some mindfulness activities can help with hearing voices. Walk around your home and pick a color. Name out loud five things of that color. Then choose another color and name four things. Then another and name three. Another and name two. Finally, pick one last color and name one thing of that color. Do this as many times as you need to.

An Image of a Voice

It can be scary to hear a voice inside or outside your head; however, it is very important to know that you are stronger than any voice. Some people find it empowering to draw an image (such as a cartoon character) to represent a voice or to name it. Putting a picture or name to the voice can make it less powerful. If you hear voices, feel free to use this space to draw what your voice might look like or to name it. If you do not hear voices, think about the critical thoughts you may experience sometimes. While this is different from hearing voices, this exercise can also help you to cope with it.

Draw the image here.

Coping With Voices

Coping strategies can help you re-focus on what matters to you and navigate through the roughest spaces. Check out some strategies here that you might like to try.

Using your voice
Sometimes activities that use our own voice out loud can help reduce the voices we hear on the inside. This includes exercises such as:

☐ Humming   ☐ Talking out loud as you write
☐ Singing   ☐ Whistling
☐ Positive self-talk out loud   ☐ Talking to another person
☐ Talking on the phone   ☐ _____

Re-focusing
Hearing voices can distract us from what matters. We can try different strategies to help us re-focus on activities that are meaningful to us such as:

☐ Writing   ☐ Building something such as a model car
☐ Playing a game
☐ Making a list of things to do   ☐ Doing a puzzle or word game
☐ Art   ☐ Doing a creative project
☐ Dancing   ☐ Acts of kindness
☐ Working on a college application   ☐ _____

Mindfulness
Mindfulness can be many things, including watching, describing, and doing. Doing a physical activity, such as walking, in a way that your focus is just on that one activity is one way to practice mindfulness.

☐ Counting breaths
☐ Deep breathing
☐ Going into nature and focusing on the sights, sounds, and feelings
☐ Examining an object up close
☐ Throwing a ball in the air
☐ Stretching
☐ Practicing yoga or tai-chi
☐ Closing your eyes and imagining a beautiful place such as a beach, castle, or wilderness

☐ _____

Connecting with others

Being alone can sometimes make voices worse. Connecting with others can help. Some ways to connect with others include:

- ☐ Attending a support group
- ☐ Reaching out to a friend or family member
- ☐ Writing a letter
- ☐ Creating a card
- ☐ Calling a phone support line such as a warm line or crisis line
- ☐ Picking up a conversation
- ☐ _____

Physical activity

Physical activity can release anxiety, encourage mindfulness, and help with voices. Activities can include:

- ☐ Walking
- ☐ Playing sports
- ☐ Spending time outdoors
- ☐ Stretching
- ☐ _____

Sensory coping

Using sensory experiences to cope is another strategy for coping with hearing voices. These can include:

Sound

- ☐ Listening to music
- ☐ Drumming or tapping
- ☐ Playing a musical instrument
- ☐ Listening to nature sounds
- ☐ _____

Vision

- ☐ Looking at an encouraging picture or affirmation
- ☐ Taking time to find a color or picture on the wall that you like
- ☐ Looking at a picture of a supportive person or animal in your life
- ☐ Coloring

☐ Drawing
☐ Making a collage

☐ _____

Touch

☐ Using lotion on your hands and noticing how this feels
☐ Fidgeting with something like a guitar pick or fidget spinner
☐ Taking a shower or bath

☐ _____

Smell

☐ Going outside and noticing appealing smells such as a flower or rain
☐ Smelling an unlit candle
☐ Smelling lotion
☐ Seeking out scents connected with positive memories (e.g., if you link up the smell of sunscreen with good times at the beach, you could smell some sunscreen)

☐ _____

Taste

☐ Having a piece of candy or another treat with a stronger taste such as mint
☐ Enjoying something with a comforting taste, such as tea
☐ Trying a taste that you associate with a positive memory (e.g., if you associate the taste and smell of popcorn with positive memories of the movies, this may be a taste to seek out)

☐ _____

Amplifying Your Own Voice

At a time in my life when I found my own mind very loud, I remember listening to an audiobook called Radical Compassion *by Tara Brach. In the book, she talked about how you could be your own best friend. To me at the time, that sounded impossible. How could I be my own best friend with this constant chatter in my head about what a bad person I am? But she was right. Rather than spending so much time shouting at the voices or trying to block them out, I began using my own voice. I talked to myself the way I would talk to someone I care about. I used a mantra of "we're good" when I felt overwhelmed. I asked myself what I needed when the thoughts were hard to ignore, and I talked myself through the steps (sometimes aloud and sometimes in my head) to do what I needed to do. All of this helped me remember that I am in control and that the voices do not get to say what kind of a person I am.*

Hearing voices can be extremely distressing. When hearing voices, you may feel urges to try to drown out the voices—for example, by hiding your ears with a hoodie or putting on headphones. It can also be tempting to talk under your breath or even shout back at the voices. There is nothing wrong with using these strategies, especially if you find these helpful in relieving your distress and moving toward your valued goals. Still, there is another strategy for coping with voices: using your own voice.

Your own voice is powerful and can help ground you. You can cultivate this tool through strategies such as positive self-talk, mantras, and even remembering kind things others have said to you. Sometimes talking out loud especially can override the voices. Always remember, at the end of the day, your own voice matters most.

Many people worry about the stigma of talking about their voices and so might think they need to hide their experiences. This can lead you to feel alone. In several communities and health clinics, groups exist where people can share their experiences of hearing voices with each other. This is another way of using your own voice to cope with voices.

Mantras

A mantra is a message you create for yourself that will remind you of what matters most or help you to ground in tough times. You can repeat a mantra to yourself, or create reminders of your mantra to encourage you throughout the day. Some people carry a mantra on a card, keychain, or painted rock. Other people use a picture to pair with their mantra.

Check boxes of the mantras which you most relate to and/or create your own below.

- ☐ I can
- ☐ Breathe
- ☐ All I have to deal with is now
- ☐ I always make it
- ☐ I am not my illness
- ☐ I am more than voices
- ☐ This will pass
- ☐ People care about me
- ☐ I am safe

- ☐ _____
- ☐ _____
- ☐ _____

Take one of the mantras you selected and write it on a piece of paper. Place it somewhere you will see it every day.

Self-Compassion

Self-compassion is a way of showing yourself the same kindness you would anyone you love, especially during times of difficulty.

Think of this: If a friend told you they were hearing voices, what would you say to them?

_____

_____

_____

_____

_____

If you hear voices, what do you tell yourself about it?

_____

_____

_____

_____

_____

Compassion is a light in dark times. Often, we are kinder to others than ourselves. Self-compassion is a way to hold a little light for yourself. Self-compassion is broken into three parts: mindfulness (being in the moment), common humanity (knowing that others deal with what we deal with), and self-kindness (showing yourself love). It takes many forms including good self-care (such as using stress shields regularly) and talking to yourself kindly.

Did you know that as many as one in ten people will hear a voice or voices within their lifetime? That is a lot of people. What is it like for you to know that so many people share this experience?

_____

_____

_____

_____

_____

One way to practice self-compassion is by remembering how alike we are. Read this passage aloud or in your mind:

Like me, other people have good times
Like me, other people struggle
Like me, some other people hear voices
Like me, other people are recovering

One final way to practice self-compassion is through "cheerleading" or saying encouraging things to yourself. This is not the same as telling yourself things that are very positive or which you don't believe. However, it is a sort of pep talk you give to yourself.

How can you cheerlead yourself through your experience of hearing voices?

_____

_____

_____

_____

_____

_____

_____

_____

_____

_____

13

Beliefs That Get in the Way

There came a time in my life when I felt very depressed. I thought of myself as evil, that anyone I came close to would be sorry. So, I started isolating myself. I also sensed that I must be so bad that even God would hate me. It got confusing. I felt so sure of it. The worst part was that I did not think I could tell anyone about this. I felt worthless and feared sharing my problems would just make their lives worse. Hadn't I been enough of a burden? But these things I believed, while they felt so real, were not true. I am not evil. God does not hate me. I am not worthless. Most of all, when I get anywhere near this mind state, sharing my thoughts with another person is essential to maintaining my wellness, and I am committed to that.

Our beliefs about things tend to change throughout our lives. Can you think of a food that you didn't like ten years ago that you do now? What we think also changes how we act and feel. If you believe that you are a chess master, you will probably feel a lot more confident before a chess tournament than if you think that you are terrible at chess!

Sometimes we have beliefs that get in the way. When a person becomes very stuck in a belief that is harmful to them, or that is not true, that belief is called a delusion. The most common belief of this kind is called paranoia. Paranoia is a type of belief where you feel that a person or people want or are going to create bad things for you. It is common, affecting as many as one in ten people at some point during their lifetime. Sometimes paranoia can also give you a sense that you are being watched, monitored, or followed. It is often a very upsetting experience.

Some people experience a feeling that the people close to them might be talking behind their back or planning to harm them. Other people have paranoia about the government or other large groups of people, like a workplace or pharmacy. It is often difficult to tell for sure if these beliefs are true or not. Still, when you are experiencing a delusion, that belief takes center stage in your mind and can get in the way of doing the things that matter to you.

Other types of delusions involve grand ideas such as that you have millions of dollars or are on a secret mission with the president. While, at first, these beliefs have a cheery tone, when you get very fixated on these thoughts, it can make it hard to live your life. You may find yourself making choices that you otherwise would never make. If you have experienced a delusion, please know that you are not alone.

Talking to an adult such as a parent or mental health professional about your beliefs can be a first step to getting help. Many people who struggle with delusions have had well-meaning people brush them off when they share their concerns or say something reassuring like "You know that's not real." It can make you feel unheard. If someone is willing to hear you out, it can go a long way toward reminding you that you are not alone in this.

Mental health professionals have training in how to help you express what is going on for you and explore how your beliefs are helping or hurting you in moving toward what is important to you. They are not here to judge you or tell you what is true or not. Therapy can give you a space to work on paranoia and other beliefs that get in the way.

Helpful Beliefs

Our beliefs change how we feel, act, and experience life. Have you ever held any of these common beliefs that tend to help people feel better and act in ways that move toward their goals?

☐ I can learn new things
☐ I am likeable
☐ I might not always succeed but that doesn't mean I am a failure
☐ I am more than my diagnosis
☐ I am strong
☐ I am not alone
☐ I can trust these people:

_____

_____

_____

☐ I can grow and change

☐ _____

☐ _____

How do/did these beliefs make your life better?

_____

_____

_____

_____

Have you ever had any beliefs such as:

☐ I cannot trust anyone
☐ People or groups of people want bad things to happen to me
☐ People are talking about me behind my back
☐ People who are against me are stronger than I am
☐ I am alone
☐ No one likes me

If you have had beliefs like this, please know that while these beliefs are powerful, you are stronger than your beliefs. Talking to someone about your belief can help.

Challenging Questions for Fear and Paranoia

Depression convinced me I was evil. At times, I had turned against myself. I would re-examine over and over all the mistakes I have made in life. It wouldn't stop there, though. I would get a sense that people around me must not like me because I would be so convinced that I am not a good person. Even there, it would not stop. I would imagine every way that people could get back at me and I would worry non-stop. I experienced paranoia. Paranoia led to isolation. Isolation led to worsening depression. Today, I can catch that pattern before it starts. When I get depressed, I know I am at risk for the same way of thinking. I recognize it quickly and work through it. If it pops up, I look at the evidence. I know that I have made some mistakes in life—everyone has—but I also care deeply about others and do my best to live my values. I am not at the mercy of my thoughts or my depression.

Most people experience fears about what others might be thinking about them or feel distrust at times. For some, these beliefs can get in the way of moving toward our goals and values. Asking challenging questions is one way to examine these beliefs and consider the evidence.

Sometimes beliefs that get in the way feel so true. Still, just because something feels true, that doesn't mean it is true. Challenging questions are a way to test out what we believe to see if it matches the facts. Because it is tough to keep track of questions in our minds when we are testing something out, writing down responses can help us sort out what we have evidence for and what we don't.

Sometimes you can check in to see if your belief is true. If you think someone could be mad at you, you could ask them. Other times, there is no easy way to check in on it. If there is someone you trust, asking for their thoughts on the matter can also be helpful. This is called reality checking.

Reality checking and challenging questions are ways to help you take a neutral view of a belief.

Reality Checking and Challenging Questions

Name an unhelpful thought.

_____

Why might this thought be true?

_____
_____
_____
_____
_____
_____
_____

Is there another possible explanation?

_____
_____
_____
_____
_____
_____
_____

Why might this thought not be true?

_____
_____
_____
_____
_____
_____
_____

What would you say to a friend who thought this?

_____
_____
_____
_____
_____
_____
_____

What thought might be more helpful?

_____

_____

Negative Symptoms

What They Are and What You Can Do About Them

There was a time when every day felt the same. I had fallen away from friends and family. Even when I was around others, it felt as if there was this invisible glass between me and everyone else—like I was disconnected. I slept all the time and had zero energy. I acted "quiet," but I did not want to disappear. I started writing just one thing I wanted to do every day. I started being around people even when I didn't "feel" it. I listened to music that meant something to me. Little by little, the sparkles of life seemed to come back for me. It wasn't all at once, but I began to feel like me again.

There are two main types of psychosis symptoms—positive and negative. Positive symptoms are the more noticeable symptoms of psychosis, such as paranoia and hearing voices. Still, while not as loud as positive symptoms, negative symptoms hinder people from moving toward their aspirations at least as much.

You might be thinking: Aren't all symptoms "negative"? Negative symptoms are those which cause us to lose something we used to have—like having less motivation, less interest in social things, feeling emotion less vividly, and having less energy. In contrast, positive symptoms add something on to your experience that could be distressing, such as hallucinations or unusual beliefs.

Some common negative symptoms include:

- having less motivation
- not wanting to be around others
- having less energy than you used to
- feeling like your emotions are flat
- showing less facial expression than you used to
- taking longer to get started on tasks
- feeling less interested in things.

The good news is that the impact of negative symptoms can be reduced by taking small steps toward identifying your interests and moving toward those. In addition, expressive acts like art, music, and movement can help raise your energy, motivation, and sense of connection to help you combat negative symptoms.

Think of it like this. Have you ever lit a campfire? A small spark will light a larger spark and eventually you have a campfire. The same is true for emotions, energy, and motivation. Since your mental health change, it might be harder to engage in things that give that spark. Still, even small steps can create a spark that can then build a bigger spark.

Drawing an Emotion

Listen to a piece of music that you have related to in the past, or which you relate to now. While you listen, draw within this circle a reflection of the emotions and experiences that come up for you. Don't worry about creating an image you want to share with someone else or hang on the wall. The purpose of this exercise is just to get more in tune with your emotional experience when you listen to this piece of music. You can choose colors, patterns, lines, or images that show what you are experiencing inside as you hear the music.

Charging up Your Motivation

Each of us is motivated by different things. What follows is a list of things that might spark your drive. Check off items that you would be willing to try in order to lift your motivation or which you have found to lift your motivation in the past.

- ☐ Being with other people
- ☐ Doing something creative
- ☐ Checking in with a mentor
- ☐ Doing something kind for someone else
- ☐ Listening to music
- ☐ Breaking my goals into small pieces
- ☐ Learning more about my role models
- ☐ Reminding myself why something is meaningful to me
- ☐ Spending time in nature
- ☐ Having a clear goal

- ☐ _____

Revisit this list when you find yourself struggling to get started with something or to move toward goals. It can take time to get your motivation back up, but small steps each day can make a huge difference! Keep trying!

Putting the Magnifying Glass on Positive Emotions

Taking time to intentionally appreciate the good things in life is another way to enhance positive emotions. Often, we may focus more on the bad things than the good things. By taking time to zoom in on the good things, we are able to appreciate these better.

Think of three "good deeds" that others have done for you. This can be something like a time a teacher stayed behind in class to help you catch up, a friend who has "been there," or a time someone returned your wallet. Make a list of these.

1. _____
2. _____
3. _____

Now, try to think of other "good things." This can be current good things in your life such as a holiday you are looking forward to or how you are enjoying the colors changing on the leaves. It could also be something like a pet, a time you remember someone showing kindness to someone else, or a favorite food. Don't overthink it. Just write what comes to mind.

1. _____
2. _____
3. _____
4. _____
5. _____
6. _____
7. _____
8. _____
9. _____
10. _____

TRY THIS
Appreciation challenge
Choose one thing you could enjoy. This could be as small as looking for shapes in clouds or as big as reaching out to someone important to you for a conversation. Take time to really enjoy just doing this one thing. You might have expectations for how things should turn out—for example, if checking out clouds, you might expect a certain color of cloud. But try to let go of expectations and appreciate whatever shows up. If you are struggling to think of something to try, check out the next activity.

Little Good Things

Below are some suggestions of little good things you can try. Tick those that you've enjoyed already or that you'd like to try, and add any suggestions of your own.

- ☐ Watching a favorite TV show
- ☐ Having a pleasant conversation
- ☐ Reading
- ☐ Watching the sunset
- ☐ Flying a kite
- ☐ Going for a walk
- ☐ Looking closely at a color you like
- ☐ Painting
- ☐ Drawing
- ☐ Swimming
- ☐ Enjoying the weather
- ☐ Listening to music
- ☐ Looking at the stars
- ☐ Learning about something you enjoy
- ☐ Smelling a candle
- ☐ Enjoying a shower
- ☐ Listening to music
- ☐ Listening to birds or nature sounds
- ☐ Enjoying lotion

☐ _____

☐ _____

☐ _____

Part 4

THRIVING WITH OTHER MENTAL HEALTH SYMPTOMS

16

Keeping Focus

Distractibility has been a lifelong thing for me. Depression brings it to the next level. It makes it hard to concentrate and finish tasks, and everyday stuff becomes a million times harder to do. As a teen, I thought it meant I must be slow or not as intelligent as other people, but I learned later that this is a common problem for people with my condition. Showing myself kindness, accompanied by adjustments like writing things down and color-coding my planner, has helped a lot.

Losing things like your keys or finding yourself distractible sometimes is normal. If you find yourself struggling with your thoughts to a point that gets in the way of your life, you may be dealing with cognitive symptoms. These are mental health symptoms related to thinking, concentration, memory, and speech. Difficulties like these can be frustrating and discouraging.

Thought-based symptoms, also called "cognitive symptoms," are common symptoms of a variety of mental health challenges, including psychosis, depression, mania, anxiety, and others. Problems like these can also be caused by physical health challenges, substance use, and stress.

Most people with cognitive symptoms find that some areas of their thinking are affected while others work fine. Some people experiencing symptoms find that it is harder to think of the right words (word-finding difficulties), but they may still do well with things like solving a maze or a puzzle in a video game.

Having cognitive symptoms does not mean that you are any less intelligent. It is important to be kind to yourself when you notice these difficulties. Strategies such as using a notebook to assist your memory or keeping things (like your phone or wallet) consistently in the same place are ways to help you cope. Knowing which cognitive symptoms you experience and letting your providers know can also assist them to help you with these.

Research shows that, for some, a specific structured intervention called Cognitive Enhancement Therapy (CET) can improve these symptoms (Eack *et al.* 2009). This involves working through brain exercises with a therapist or on a computer. If you are interested in learning more, talk to your clinician about what is available.

Your Cognitive Symptoms

Check off any cognitive symptoms listed that you relate to.

- ☐ Losing things
- ☐ Trouble finishing tasks
- ☐ Trouble finding words for things
- ☐ Forgetting names easily
- ☐ Difficulty concentrating
- ☐ Finding others cannot understand what words I am saying
- ☐ A sense that my thoughts are super slowed down
- ☐ A sense that my thoughts are super sped up
- ☐ Losing my train of thought a lot
- ☐ Forgetting things easily
- ☐ Trouble reading facial expressions
- ☐ Difficulty recognizing faces

- ☐ _____
- ☐ _____
- ☐ _____

Remember that many of the challenges listed above are normal human experiences; however, if you find these are getting in the way of your daily life, it may be worthwhile trying some of the adaptive strategies listed in the next activity.

Your Adaptive Strategies

Check off adaptive strategies you would be willing to try to improve your cognition.

- ☐ Practicing brain games
- ☐ Putting things like my wallet and phone in the same place every day
- ☐ Writing myself sticky notes to remember things I need to finish
- ☐ Setting reminders on my phone
- ☐ Keeping a planner
- ☐ Giving myself kindness for my challenges
- ☐ Knowing that these are common symptoms and do not mean I am stupid or not trying hard enough
- ☐ Keeping a calendar
- ☐ Practicing repeating another person's name in conversation to make it more likely for me to remember: for example, "Hey, I'm John." "Nice to meet you, John."
- ☐ Checking in with others to see if they understand what I am saying
- ☐ Purposely slowing down what I am doing so I can keep better track of things
- ☐ Keeping a notebook
- ☐ Practicing reading facial expressions

- ☐ _____
- ☐ _____
- ☐ _____

17

Sleep Problems

Sleep has been difficult for me throughout my life. The tricky thing about sleep for me is that sleep problems are both a symptom and a trigger for my symptoms. I am very protective of my sleep. I know that if I do not go to bed and get up around the same time each day, I am likely to struggle.

Most people know that sleep affects mood; however, you might not know that sleep is also key to learning, remembering things, being able to think clearly, and maintaining your physical health. Lack of sleep can be a powerful trigger for mental health symptoms, especially psychosis, mania or mood highs, and depression. Sleep deprivation can cause psychosis even in people who do not otherwise have a mental health condition (Petrovsky *et al.* 2014).

Still, getting enough sleep is not easy for everyone. Compared to those without mental health issues, young adults who live with mental health conditions are more likely to have trouble with sleep. This could range from sleeping too much, not being able to fall asleep, or finding that their natural sleep rhythms do not fall in line with those that society has imposed on them.

Practicing healthy sleep hygiene is one thing you can do to help improve your sleep rhythms. While these strategies take practice and might not always be what you want to do in the moment, over time they can help you get good rest. In turn, this can improve your mental health and overall quality of life.

In addition, if you notice significant sleep difficulties or find that your sleep issues are worsening your symptoms, do not hesitate to discuss this with your treatment team. Psychotherapies such as Cognitive Behavioral Therapy for Insomnia and medical treatments can help to ease sleep issues. Recognizing your sleep patterns and how these relate to your patterns of mental health symptoms could also provide valuable insight as you seek control of your mental health symptoms.

Improving Your Sleep

Shade in the moons representing strategies that you already use to improve your sleep hygiene.

Circle ones you would be willing to try.

Go to bed at the same time
each night

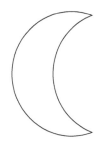

Get up at the same time
each morning

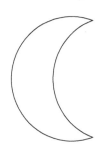

Do the same thing every night before bed
(e.g., reading or taking a shower)

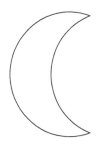

Don't use caffeine
before bed

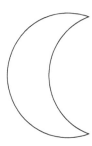

Keep away from electronics
one hour before bed

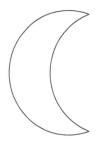

Sleep with phone away
from bed

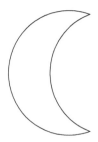

What to Do When You Can't Sleep

Even if you are using good sleep hygiene practices, there may still be times you have trouble falling asleep. These are some things you can do which may help on nights when it is difficult to fall asleep. Shade in ones you would be willing to try.

Get out of bed and
do something

Get my things ready
for the next day

Imagine beautiful
scenery

Listen to music

Practice deep
breathing

Say a calming word
or phrase to myself

18

Letting Go of Addictions

For a period, there were very few things that I enjoyed doing. I felt down all the time. I spent a lot of time scrolling through social media. It was fun at first and helped me connect to friends. Yet, in time, I found that even when I was physically with other people, my mind would be thinking about what was going on online. I watched other people live their lives instead of fully living my own. It affected the things that matter to me in life, like showing up for those around me. I started practicing leaving my phone on the charger more unless I needed it. I still like social media, but it no longer blocks me from being present or gets in the way of things that matter to me.

If you are tempted to use substances or other addictive behaviors to help yourself feel better, you are not the only one. Many people do. Unfortunately, people with mental health conditions are much more likely than those without to suffer from addictions (Kessler 2004).

While it is true that some people report that addictive behaviors help them feel better in the short term, in the long term these can derail your goals and harm your health. Rather than relieving stress, addiction tricks you into feeling less stressed in the short run by giving you even more to worry about when all is said and done. Cannabis use, in particular, has been linked with the development of psychosis in some people (Arseneault *et al.* 2004).

Of course, substance use is not the only challenge of this kind that people struggle with. Things like gambling, too much time on technology, eating problems, overspending, and self-harm are also popular ways to try to feel better in the short term, which ultimately lead to more suffering in the long term. Of course, this is not an exhaustive list. There are hundreds of addictive behaviors that people struggle with.

If you are struggling with challenges like these, know you are not alone. Having an addiction is nothing to be ashamed of, and help is available. It is also okay if you aren't sure if you want to stop or even if you don't know for sure that you have an addiction. Talking to your treatment team about your addictive behaviors can help you consider your options, as well as reduce the harm done by these difficulties.

The Many Faces of Addiction

Are there any challenges you struggle with that are causing you more problems in the long term?

- ☐ Overuse of social media
- ☐ Eating challenges
- ☐ Self-harm
- ☐ Substance use
- ☐ Overuse of gaming
- ☐ Overspending

☐ _____

☐ _____

☐ _____

On a scale of 1–10, how open are you to discussing this challenge with your treatment team?

_____

What would help you feel more comfortable discussing it?

- ☐ Bringing a support person with me
- ☐ Writing about it first
- ☐ Knowing that I would not be judged

☐ _____

☐ _____

☐ _____

Your Life in Five Years

Imagine yourself in five years if you continue to engage in your identified addictive behavior. What would your life look like? Your relationships? Would you be working or in school? Draw a picture of this.

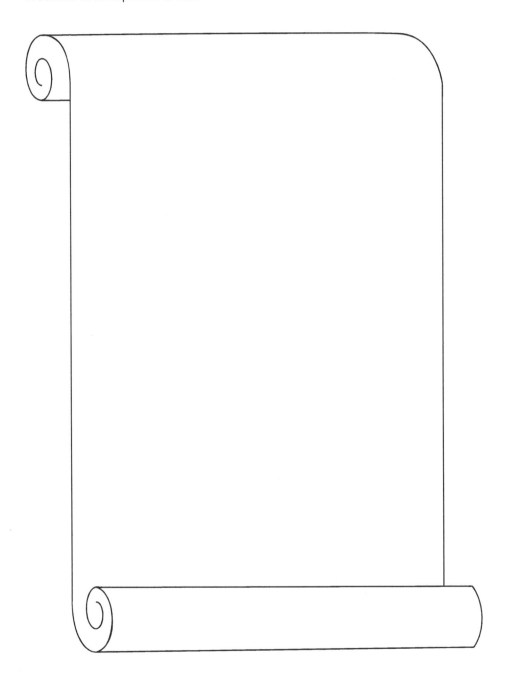

Now, imagine yourself five years from now if you stop your identified addictive behavior. What would your life look like? Your relationships? Would you be working or in school? Draw a picture of this.

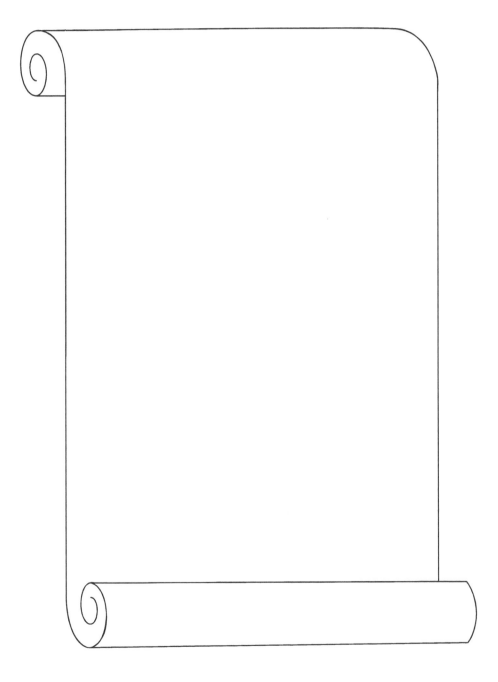

The Pros and Cons of Addiction

What would be the biggest positives of working on your addiction?

- ☐ Improving my relationships
- ☐ Living my values
- ☐ Meeting work goals
- ☐ Feeling in control
- ☐ Knowing I can cope
- ☐ Meeting educational goals
- ☐ Improving my physical health
- ☐ Improving my mental health

☐ _____

☐ _____

☐ _____

What would be the biggest negatives of working on your addiction?

- ☐ Letting go of something that helps me to cope
- ☐ Not knowing if I can
- ☐ Feeling less in control
- ☐ Missing my "highs"

☐ _____

☐ _____

☐ _____

How can you work around these barriers?

- ☐ Make a list of my reasons for dropping my addiction
- ☐ Ask for support
- ☐ Read or watch inspirational stories of people who have overcome addictions

☐ _____

☐ _____

☐ _____

19

Action Against Depression

When I feel depressed, sometimes it is difficult to do the stuff I have to do, let alone the things I want to do. I want to sleep and be left alone. That's it. Trouble is, those are choices that allow my depression to grow worse. I have found that sometimes just taking a step outside or doing one fun thing often gives me some happiness when I am down even if I do not think it will. This is what I can do to work against depression. It does help.

Depression is an expert at shapeshifting. Sometimes it can show up loud—as sadness and irritation. Other times it is more subtle—a feeling of not wanting to do things. Depression can pull the joy out of the positive things in life. Sometimes depression is biological and part of an illness. Depression can also be a normal reaction to painful life events.

Like any other health condition, depression is not your fault. Depression is not the same as feeling sorry for yourself or having a bad attitude. It is a complex, often biologically linked disorder.

If you feel depressed, it is important to let your treatment team know. Depression can convince you that there is no hope and you will never feel better. Nothing could be further from the truth. Depression is very treatable. With assistance, your spirits can lift again, you can re-engage in the things you love, and you can begin enjoying life again.

A major difficulty that some people experience during depression is thoughts of suicide and self-harm. If this is something that you are struggling with, please know that you are not alone. Many have been where you are and rediscovered a sense of hope. This said, you cannot keep this symptom a secret. If you are having thoughts about harming yourself, please reach out to your treatment providers right away.

One of the main tools to battle depression is behavioral activation. This is a fancy term for getting active—doing things that give you a sense of accomplishment and/or that you enjoy. Sometimes this may be the same. For example, you might both enjoy writing poetry and feel a sense of accomplishment when you finish a poem. It is okay for these things to be different as well—for example, you might enjoy going to an ice cream parlour, but it might not give you much of a sense of accomplishment.

Behavior activation is a strategy of balancing these actions, taking small steps toward a more active life. In addition, behavior activation is ideally crafted around your strengths and values, showing up as something specifically meaningful to you.

Your Symptoms of Depression

Do you experience any of these symptoms of depression?

- ☐ Not wanting to do things you normally enjoy
- ☐ Feeling sad
- ☐ Feeling less hope for the future
- ☐ Trouble falling asleep or staying asleep
- ☐ Wanting to sleep a lot
- ☐ Feeling less energy
- ☐ Eating less
- ☐ Eating more
- ☐ Trouble concentrating
- ☐ Feeling slowed down
- ☐ Feeling more irritable or annoyed with people
- ☐ Withdrawing from other people

- ☐ _____
- ☐ _____
- ☐ _____

If you are experiencing difficulties such as these, please let your treatment team know. Depression is treatable.

Fun Things

Take a look at these enjoyable activities. Put a checkmark next to any you would be open to trying.

- ☐ Playing a video game
- ☐ Listening to music
- ☐ Photography
- ☐ Designing an original character
- ☐ Cooking
- ☐ Taking a walk
- ☐ Meeting with friends
- ☐ Exploring a new place
- ☐ Visiting a park
- ☐ Walking around the mall
- ☐ Feeding birds
- ☐ Riding a bicycle
- ☐ Visiting a family member
- ☐ Getting nails done
- ☐ Going hiking
- ☐ Getting a haircut
- ☐ Whistling
- ☐ Brewing coffee or tea
- ☐ Fishing
- ☐ Going to a coffee shop
- ☐ Listening to the birds
- ☐ Feeding fish
- ☐ Reading
- ☐ Going to a gym
- ☐ Playing a game
- ☐ Going skating
- ☐ Giving someone a compliment
- ☐ Playing an instrument
- ☐ Dancing
- ☐ Going to a community event
- ☐ Going thrift shopping
- ☐ Learning something new
- ☐ Journaling
- ☐ _____
- ☐ _____
- ☐ _____

Things That Give You a Sense of Accomplishment

Take a look at these activities that can give you a sense of accomplishment. Put a checkmark next to the ones that you would be willing to try out.

- ☐ Emailing or calling a place I could volunteer
- ☐ Caring for an animal
- ☐ Joining a club
- ☐ Making a game
- ☐ Volunteering
- ☐ Working on a class assignment
- ☐ Looking at prospective colleges
- ☐ Learning a new skill
- ☐ Working on a project
- ☐ Writing
- ☐ Cooking
- ☐ Photography
- ☐ Completing a college application
- ☐ Making my bed
- ☐ Taking a shower
- ☐ Getting a haircut
- ☐ Cleaning out my car
- ☐ Writing a goal list
- ☐ Learning a magic trick
- ☐ Reading
- ☐ Talking to a mentor
- ☐ Creating a vision board
- ☐ Exercising
- ☐ Attending an appointment
- ☐ Attending a support group or class
- ☐ Helping a friend or family member
- ☐ Visiting a gym
- ☐ Fixing something
- ☐ Saying hello to someone
- ☐ Writing a letter or email
- ☐ Paying a bill
- ☐ Signing up for a class
- ☐ _____
- ☐ _____
- ☐ _____

BINGO Challenge

Choose activities from the above two lists and write on your choices. See if you can get BINGO by doing the activities and marking them off.

Riding Waves of Anxiety

Anxiety to me tends to feel like an anvil hanging over my head. It is hard to relax; I shake. My impulse is to get out of the situation. I used to hide from my anxiety. Today, I would not call my anxiety a "friend"; however, I know that I do not have to hide from it anymore. I do not enjoy it, but I am not afraid of it. It is something I know I can ride through when I need to.

Anxiety is not all bad. Before you throw this book across the room, hear me out. Anxious scanning and quick reactions helped our ancestors to survive threats like tigers, avalanches, and attacks from unfriendly others. It gears us up to fight or flee in dangerous situations.

Chances are, lions and tigers are far from your top anxiety triggers. Still, no doubt there has been at least one time in your life when anxiety gave you a hand. You might have been anxious about a test, so you studied and got a good grade as a result. Perhaps there was a time you shook your shoes before putting them on your feet, knowing a spider could be hiding there, and watched a little hairy eight-legged creature fall out. Even today, some level of anxiety is a good thing.

You can think of anxiety as being like the "check engine" light on a car. It tells you that something is wrong, but it doesn't always tell you what. Sometimes you know right away what is wrong (like when you see a venomous snake near you), and in that case, anxiety is doing its job (giving you the energy to get away if you need to or take other steps to address the problem). Anxiety's best "jam" is preparing us to deal with threats outside our heads.

Sometimes that "check engine" light flickers when you are at no risk at all. This can show up as a looming feeling that something is not right, feeling on edge, worrying, or sudden attacks of physical symptoms. Clinical anxiety is like this. You can think of it as a faulty "check engine" light. In addition, most threats we deal with in our modern world are social and emotional. Of course, these are still real dangers. Still, the old-school action urges of anxiety rarely help.

Even when there is no physical threat, your anxiety likely will tell you to do what it would in the case of a tiger—to fight off your threat (with irritability or anger) or run off and avoid the situation. In these situations, hiding or lashing out might only carry you further away from what matters to you.

Anxiety will lie to you and tell you things like:

- ☒ If you don't worry, something bad will happen.
- ☒ You can't handle anxiety.
- ☒ Anxiety can physically hurt you.
- ☒ If you are anxious, you have to leave the situation.

None of this is true. Anxiety tells you that you can't handle it. It says that unless you get out of the situation, you will feel horrible, or something bad will happen.

Anxiety is quite the bully!

But you don't have to listen to it.

Here's what anxiety won't tell you:

- ☑ No matter what, you won't be anxious forever.
- ☑ You can ride through the sensations of anxiety and go back to what you enjoy.
- ☑ You can't die from a panic attack.
- ☑ Most things you worry about never happen.
- ☑ Avoiding things that make you anxious makes your anxiety stronger.

Anxiety tends to give us an urge to avoid; however, avoiding situations that make us anxious tends to strengthen our anxiety over time and keeps us from enjoying things that are important to us. Remember, we only get anxious about things that matter to us! You can think of your anxiety as waves. When you are feeling anxious, the anxiety will naturally grow and then slow down, just like a wave. You can ride the waves.

Avoidance is like getting out of the ocean. But the ocean is beautiful! Over time, avoidance causes anxiety to get worse as your life gets smaller.

Situations that make us anxious tend to correspond to our hopes, dreams, and loves. Another option is to ride the waves of anxiety and focus on doing what you want to do while remembering that anxiety cannot truly hurt you.

TRY THIS

3-2-1

Grounding is an exercise to help you get back into the moment and ride the waves of emotion. A simple grounding exercise is 3-2-1. It's simple:

  3...name three things you see
  2....name two things you hear
  1...name one thing you feel.

Do this as many times as you need to. Focus in depth on the colors of what you see, the pitches of the sounds, and the felt sense of what you feel. Describe it. This will help you ride the waves.

Your Symptoms of Anxiety

How do you experience anxiety?

- ☐ Worrying
- ☐ Trouble relaxing
- ☐ Shaking
- ☐ Heart beating fast
- ☐ Quick breathing
- ☐ Trouble falling asleep
- ☐ Numbness
- ☐ Zoning out
- ☐ Difficulty concentrating
- ☐ Difficulty catching your breath
- ☐ Wanting to leave the situation making you anxious
- ☐ Sweating a lot
- ☐ Racing thoughts
- ☐ Feeling like you might lose control
- ☐ Feeling like something bad might happen

- ☐ _____
- ☐ _____
- ☐ _____

Draw a Picture of Anxiety

It might seem strange to draw a picture of anxiety; however, sometimes creating an image of anxiety can take away some of its power. You might draw your anxiety as a creature, a person, or even a set of shapes and lines. Think about what image might reflect your anxiety best.

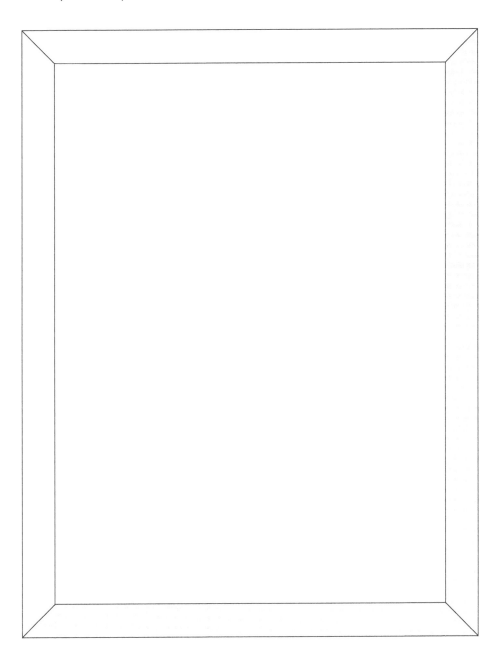

Guided Imagery

Imagine yourself lying in an ocean on an inflatable raft. You can feel the warm water below you and see beautiful patterns of blue. Maybe you can also smell the sweet smell of salt water and sunscreen. Notice how your raft rises and falls with the waves. It is relaxing in a way. You rise and fall. Up and down. You are safe.

How was this for you?

_____
_____
_____
_____
_____
_____
_____

How is dealing with anxiety like riding waves in an ocean?

_____
_____
_____
_____
_____
_____
_____

Part 5

CRISIS PLANNING

21

Creating a Crisis Plan

After my first crisis, I wanted to move on and never look back. That's not always how things work. It took three hospitalizations before what would be my last hospitalization. At 16, I attended a mental health recovery class where together we wrote a crisis plan. Creating a crisis plan gave me back control of something that I thought I could have no control over at all.

The word "crisis" often brings to mind pictures of fires, tornados, and other disasters. A crisis is a state where our resources for coping no longer meet the mountain of the stress faced. A mental health crisis is an emergency of mental health symptoms and is marked by a struggle with completing everyday tasks, strong symptoms, or thoughts to harm yourself or others.

While often upsetting, having a mental health crisis is not a failure. Recognizing that you are having a hard time and seeking help as soon as possible is key to re-balancing. Having a plan for how you would like others to help you that is written down and shared with people close to you is one way to re-empower you during a crisis and make this process as smooth as possible.

A word on hospitalization

Mental health treatment seeks to keep you in the community and out of the hospital as much as possible. Many people living with a mental health challenge never need inpatient care. Still, there may be times when your treatment team recommends a hospitalization, or when the hospital is the safest place for your treatment for a period.

Most psychiatric hospital stays are short, lasting two to seven days, with a focus on moving you out of crisis and getting you as close to your typical place of health as possible. A day in a psychiatric unit usually involves group therapy, visits with a psychiatrist or other health professionals, and meals. Some hospitals also have access to a small space outside, a gym, or a creative therapies room for art/music therapies. If you do go to a hospital, these are strategies that could help you get the most out of your visit:

- If you see a clinician outside the hospital, ask ahead of time if there is a hospital they would recommend you use if you ever need hospitalization.

While it is not always possible to see your primary psychiatrist while in hospital, admission to a hospital your provider is familiar with can sometimes help with communication.

- Know that you may not be able to keep all of your personal belongings while in hospital. The hospital may allow you to keep things like slippers, yoga-style pants with no straps, and t-shirts. Belts, things with strings (including some bras), and hygiene items that contain alcohol will probably not be allowed.
- Ask about visiting and phone hours. Unlike hospital floors for physical health, psychiatric units often have more restrictive policies for visitors and may allow you to only have visitors for one or two hours each day, or only on certain days. Knowing what days and times you will be available for visitors will make it easier for them to communicate with you.
- Be kind to those around you. Everyone goes to the hospital for a different reason. If you notice people acting in unusual ways, remember that they may be very frightened or confused.
- Keep an open mind. Be willing to learn from the groups and try the activities offered. In the hospital, you may be offered therapies you have never tried before involving music, art, or even dance. While some of it may seem silly at times, you may be surprised by what helps you or at least brightens your stay a bit.
- Ask any questions you have. Good information is empowering. Learning about your care, the medications prescribed (if you are given medication), and recommendations to avoid relapse can help you in your recovery.

Mental Health Crisis Plan

What signs might indicate that you were approaching a mental health crisis?

- ☐ Not sleeping for several nights in a row
- ☐ Desires to hurt myself
- ☐ Not being able to tell what is real and what is not
- ☐ Thoughts of wanting to harm others
- ☐ Finding my space to be getting way messier than usual
- ☐ Having urges to destroy my belongings
- ☐ Missing work or school
- ☐ Becoming very confused
- ☐ People seeming not to understand what I am saying even though it makes sense to me
- ☐ A vague feeling that I am in danger
- ☐ Feeling extremely low
- ☐ Feeling extremely high
- ☐ Eating much less than usual
- ☐ Not taking care of my personal hygiene
- ☐ _____
- ☐ _____
- ☐ _____

Who can help you if you were in a crisis?

- ☐ My psychiatrist or other prescriber
- ☐ My family member
- ☐ My friend
- ☐ My therapist
- ☐ My peer support specialist
- ☐ _____
- ☐ _____
- ☐ _____

Is there anyone you would not want to help you if you were to have a mental health crisis?

_____

_____

How can others help you if you are in a mental health crisis?

- ☐ Keep me company/not have me be alone
- ☐ Encourage me
- ☐ Help me contact my mental health providers
- ☐ Do an activity with me to help me calm down
- ☐ Take me to an Emergency Room
- ☐ Help me call a crisis line
- ☐ Remind me that I have gotten through a crisis before and am resilient
- ☐ _____
- ☐ _____
- ☐ _____

What thing do you need others *not* to do if you are in a mental health crisis?

- ☐ Yell
- ☐ Blame me or other people
- ☐ Threaten me
- ☐ Tell me if I did not _____ I would not be in this place
- ☐ Talk to other people behind my back
- ☐ Leave me alone
- ☐ Crowd me with too many people
- ☐ Ask me a lot of questions at once
- ☐ _____
- ☐ _____
- ☐ _____

If you were to have a mental health crisis, what responsibilities of yours would need to be taken care of?

- ☐ School responsibilities (e.g., letting school know if I am in need an extension on assignment deadlines due to strong symptoms or a hospitalization)
- ☐ Work responsibilities (e.g., notifying my work if I am unable to be at work)
- ☐ Animal responsibilities (e.g., having someone take care of my pets if I am in hospital or unable to look after them)
- ☐ Childcare
- ☐ _____
- ☐ _____
- ☐ _____

What is your plan for these responsibilities if you were to have a mental health crisis?

_____

_____

_____

_____

_____

If you were to have thoughts about harming yourself or others, how can you keep yourself safe?

- ☐ Reach out to my treatment provider's emergency exchange
- ☐ Present to the Emergency Room
- ☐ Connect to a crisis line or to the national suicide prevention lifeline

☐ _____

What are your reasons for living?

_____

_____

_____

_____

_____

If you are ever in crisis, what do you hope to remember?

- ☐ I can get through this
- ☐ All I have to deal with is right now
- ☐ I am loved
- ☐ I have gotten through difficult times before
- ☐ I am a good person

☐ _____ is here to help me

- ☐ I matter

☐ _____

☐ _____

☐ _____

22

After a Crisis

Coming home after each hospitalization was different, but there were a few similarities. The first was an appreciation of my freedom. I felt gratitude for things like getting to take a shower anytime I wanted. Also, I felt overwhelmed. I would be behind in school and desperately wanted to catch up. Still, concentrating on schoolwork felt impossible. I felt embarrassed. I did not want people to know I had been in hospital. But living in a small town, word gets around quick. I had to be kind to myself. I had to be on my own side. I promised myself over and over that I would recover.

After a crisis or hospitalization, a barrage of stress may greet you upon your return. You may have to deal with stressors that had affected you before or partially triggered your mental health crisis, or ongoing stress related to work, school, or relationships. Life responsibilities tend to pile up while we are unable to handle things to our best. You may have missed classes or days at work. Of course, the crisis itself also usually carries its own stress. Just going through the symptoms and treatment is exhausting and sometimes traumatic.

It's also not uncommon before and during a crisis to let go of things such as cleaning, hygiene, and checking mail. Returning to these things is overwhelming. It is okay to ask for help as you manage these stressors. In addition to picking up the pieces after a crisis, a top priority at this time is to not go back into crisis. We know that stress is a common trigger. Make it a priority to recognize early signs of stress and have a plan to tackle them.

You also may have treated people differently from how you aim to. Symptoms make it hard for us to be at our best. While having a mental health crisis is nothing to be ashamed of, depending on what happened during your experience, there may be some need for relationship repair. Be kind to yourself at this time. A mental health crisis is not your fault. Treat yourself with the same love you would after any other difficult time in your life. If you typically do not treat yourself with kindness, treat yourself as you would hope someone you care about would treat you.

As you create a plan, know it is also okay to ask for help. For example, if you need extra time to complete work or school-related tasks, you can ask if this is an option. You might also ask those around you to help with responsibilities such as caring for pets until you are feeling like yourself again.

Mental Health After-Crisis Plan

Looking back at your crisis, what is one thing you have learned ?

_____

_____

_____

_____

_____

_____

What do you need in this time?

_____

_____

_____

_____

_____

_____

What responsibilities might need tending to?

_____

_____

_____

_____

_____

_____

What is your plan for tending to these?

_____

_____

_____

_____

_____

_____

Who can help?

_____

_____

_____

_____

_____

_____

Are there any relationships that may need repair?

_____

_____

_____

_____

_____

How can you repair these?

_____

_____

_____

_____

_____

Part 6

MINDFULNESS AND DEFUSION

23

Breathing Into Stress Relief

When a therapist told me that deep breathing relieves stress, I did not believe them. I was more than willing to try, but nervousness followed me everywhere. How was changing how I breathe going to make any difference? The truth is that breathwork has changed my life in small and big ways. It gives me an extra moment to think by creating space between me and my mental experiences, to catch my feet steady on the ground and choose which way to step. That is huge, but it took time. I practice breathwork every day. It does not make my anxiety go away per se, but it keeps me from getting carried away with it.

Breathwork is a name for many exercises that use your breath to help you grab hold of the moment. One cool thing about breathwork is that you can only focus on your breath at the current point in time. When you are focused on your breath, you are in the present. Being mindful. You aren't thinking about your breath in the past or your breath in the future, just right now.

Some breathwork involves just focusing on the breath. Exercises like counting breaths or just noticing your breath without changing it sort of reel you back into the moment. It is normal during these exercises for your mind to wander at times. If this happens, notice that and then re-focus on your breath. Think of it as training a bird to fly into a cage. When the bird flies off, when your mind wanders, gently and kindly guide it back to your breath.

Other breathwork focuses on altering breath in some way. While there are many ways to do this, the most common is to slow it down. Drawing slow, deep breaths also slows down your heart rate and can help calm a racing mind. There are different ways to do this. The most common ones involve breathing in through your nose and out through your mouth, with the out-breath being longer than the in-breath. The reason for this is that the in-breath helps gear your systems up while the out-breath slows things down. Breathing in this way, and especially doing it at a slow pace, tends to calm us.

You might find breathwork comes easily for you, and if so, that's great! However, if you find that you are like most of us and become distracted when practicing breathwork, that is okay too. This is something where practice is required. A daily exercise of breathwork, especially during times when you are already calm, will give you a chance to master the skill for when you most need it.

Breath Exercises

Try these breath exercises and put a star next to the ones you find most helpful.

COUNTING BREATHS

Did you know that people take an average of 18 breaths a minute? Put a timer on for one minute and count how many you take.

BREATH AS AN ANCHOR

Think about a ship casting an anchor down to the ocean floor. Just as that anchor can hold the ship down, you can also use your breath to center yourself. Take a moment to just notice your breath.

DEEP BREATHING

Practice taking slow, deep breaths in through your nose and out through your mouth. Try to make the out breath last longer than the in breath. Start with five in, six out. After that, try six in, seven out. Finally, try seven in, eight out.

COLOR BREATHING

Imagine a color you associate with stress and a color you associate with relaxation. As you breathe in, imagine the relaxing color coming in and filling your body. As you breathe out, imagine the stress color leaving your body.

Defusion

What It Is and How It Can Help

There was a time when I felt tricked and trapped. My mind had always been my property, you know? I could decide what to think and feel. When my mental health conditions began, it felt like I lost control over that property and someone else moved in. Loud thoughts would enter my mind, and the more I tried to make them go away, the louder the thoughts got. I learned that there could be another way. I could allow the thoughts to be there, and then re-focus on what mattered to me.

Defusion is a fancy word for letting go of control of your thoughts to move toward what matters to you. This might sound like a scary idea, but the reality is that none of us can completely control our thoughts.

TRY THIS

Whatever you do, please don't think about a pizza delivery driver breakdancing on your front porch. Just don't. Don't think of that delivery driver.

What are you thinking of?

Even if you've never thought about a pizza delivery driver breakdancing on your front porch before, you are thinking of it now. And that's okay! No doubt there are thoughts you have tried to push out of your head before, and you may have learned that trying to whisk away thoughts often makes them stronger. It's not surprising, then, that you found it difficult to not think about the breakdancing delivery driver!

Now, try this: Think about a pizza delivery driver. Now think about a pizza. Pineapple, of course. Now, imagine that you are dancing through a field of flowers. Now, try to remember the last show you watched.

Isn't it amazing how quickly and effectively we are able to change the topic of our focus?

When we get fused with a thought, it overshadows everything in our minds. It is front and center stage in our minds. De-fusion is exercising our power of attention to zoom the camera lens out a bit and see the rest of the stage.

One way to think of it is like this. Sometimes we can get so caught up in our thoughts that it almost feels as if we are our thoughts. This is fusion. Defusion frees you from your thoughts. Rather than being our thoughts, defusion reminds us that we have thoughts but are separate from our thoughts.

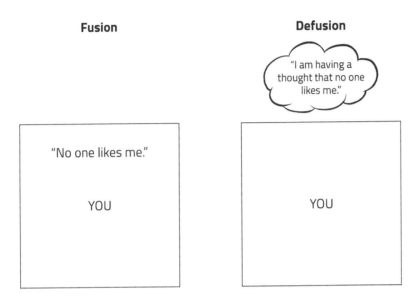

Defusion is a way of noticing our thoughts without getting stuck on them. It's like watching your thoughts move away like passing clouds. You can catch a thought and have it be there without getting wrapped up in it. If this sounds hard, it is because it is. Still, like a muscle, with exercise, it is possible to build this talent.

One way to practice defusion is simply by noticing your thoughts. This can be as small a thing as adding the words "I am noticing a thought that…." to something that comes to your mind. You are not your thoughts; you are the person noticing your thoughts. It might seem silly or extra at first; however, in the heat of the moment, we often forget to separate ourselves from our thoughts. Our thoughts blend into reality.

TRY THIS

Think about a carnival ride. Imagine it in vivid detail. What it is like to be on that ride. The feel of the seats moving up and down (or back and forth). The sounds. The sights. Isn't it amazing that we can conjure something like that up without even being there for real?

But there is a trick—our minds also sometimes use this against us. Have you ever worried so strongly about something that it felt like it was actually happening? Have you ever worried about something that did not happen? In Acceptance Commitment Therapy, the mind is called the most masterful of storytellers (a classic form of fusion). Our mind tells us stories about things all the time. Some of these stories are happening here and now. Others have happened in the past, and some will happen in the future. Most will never happen. This is the magic of our mind—to create things out of nothing.

Sometimes we get so used to a story our mind has told us that it just feels like the truth. These stories are things like "I can't do well at school," "I am a bad person," or "No one likes me." The more we repeat these things to ourselves, the truer they feel, but all of this is subjective. There are stories we have gotten very used to telling ourselves and sometimes continue to tell ourselves even when the evidence is not there or when, deep down, we don't believe them anymore.

Stories in Your Mind

In Acceptance Commitment Therapy, the mind is often called a masterful storyteller. Our minds can tell us all kinds of stories (worries, thoughts, ideas), both about things that will happen and things that never happen. In the space below, draw a storyteller and, in the bubbles, write some of the stories your mind has told you.

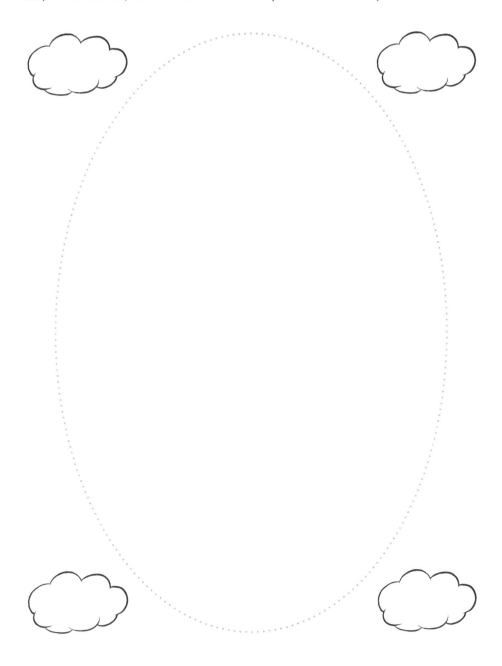

Defusion with Eagles

In a moment, close your eyes and imagine yourself standing in a field with a journal. Envision yourself looking up and noticing above you a group of beautiful eagles circling. If you can't visualize things easily, try to create a mental experience in your mind however it looks for you. Pay close attention to the awe-inspiring sight of the eagles, the sounds in this space, and, most importantly, how it feels to be in this space. As you are doing this, thoughts are bound to come up such as "Am I doing this right" or "What am I going to eat later?" If this happens, write the thought on the paper and watch as an eagle comes down and grasps the paper and returns to the circling. If another thought comes up, the same thing will happen. Enjoy this for about two minutes.

How was this for you?

_____

_____

_____

_____

_____

_____

_____

_____

_____

_____

Ways to Practice Defusion

Here is a list of ideas for practicing defusion. Check the boxes of those you would be open to trying.

- ☐ Visualizing my thoughts as words on a chalkboard
- ☐ Focusing on an image in my mind and then changing things about it—such as changing the color scheme, adding lights, or imagining a cartoon character entering the scene
- ☐ Noticing my thoughts—for example, thinking I am noticing I am having a thought that _____
- ☐ Thinking of my mind as a masterful storyteller
- ☐ Envisioning myself holding a bundle of balloons representing my thoughts and letting go of those balloons one at a time

TRY THIS

One final way to practice defusion is by naming a thought or category of thoughts. For example, many people find themselves getting into "what if" thinking, or streams of thought that start with "what if" such as "What if my car won't start?" "What if I fail the test?" "What if the zombies attack?" By calling these thoughts out as "what if" thoughts, you can recognize them more quickly and dismiss them if you wish. Other names people give these kinds of thoughts include runaway thoughts, rabbit holes, worries, or mind drifting.

Name a type of thought you experience. For example, if you sometimes get into spirals of "what ifs," you might call this "what if thinking." If you find yourself sometimes jumping to a great catastrophe in terms of your fears, you might call these "runaway thoughts." Choose whatever words feel best for you.

Walking Mindfulness

I kept hearing about mindfulness and how good it was for finding a sense of peace and grounding. For me, it felt impossible to sit still and focus for long. I would be restless, and my mind would race. But I also remembered how I felt in the summers when I would stay in a cabin with family, go hiking, and fish. I thought that was my version of mindfulness. Today, I still consider time in nature to be a powerful means of meditation.

Mindfulness is a catchy term for a simple idea: having your body and your mind in the same place at once. Often we go through the day and find ourselves caught up in thoughts, especially about the past or future. It is as if our bodies are in one place, but our minds are somewhere else.

Mindfulness is about breaking through that to access the moment. Often we find ourselves judging—thinking about things that *should* be or getting lost in our expectations. Mindfulness is also about suspending those expectations of what could be and just taking in the whole of what is right now.

Many people think of mindfulness as sitting cross-legged on the floor, inching toward enlightenment. Certain types of mindfulness involve practices such as this, but not all do. Some find mindfulness in set mindfulness practices such as counting breaths or a body scan. Others find mindfulness by focusing all their attention on a piece of music or a nature walk. There is no right or wrong here. The key is to focus on just one thing at a time—to have your body and mind in sync. If you want to walk mindfully, just walk. If you want to listen mindfully, just listen.

Expect your mind to chatter on and distract you at times! Our minds are fantastic at creating noise, and that's okay. Practicing mindfulness means bringing your attention back to your focus over and over. So, for example, if you are going on a mindful walk and have a thought like "I am so out of shape" or "I should check my phone," you can choose whether to engage with that thought. Mindfulness is noticing a thought and then re-focusing to the best of your ability on what you are doing. It is a talent that takes time to grow, and everyone loses focus sometimes when learning mindfulness. Still, with time, engaging in mindfulness can help you focus more sharply, improve your health, and increase your enjoyment in the everyday.

What follows is a specific mindfulness activity: walking mindfulness.

Walking Mindfulness

Choose a space to take a walk. This could be a walk through your neighborhood, a park, or a space that is special to you such as a garden. As you walk, notice:

- what you see
- what you hear
- what you feel
- any smells.

Are there plants in your space? What colors do you notice? How does it feel to be in this space? Also notice what it feels like to be in your body in this space. Notice the movement of your legs and arms as you walk. What it feels like to breathe the air. How the air tastes.

If you notice your mind moving to something else, know that this is completely normal! It is an opportunity to practice building strength in re-focusing, which is an invaluable skill.

How was this for you?

_____

_____

_____

_____

_____

_____

_____

_____

Part 7

YOUR STORY

26

A Kaleidoscope of Emotions

For a time, I divided my life into two parts: before my first hospitalization and after. It felt like my life stopped in a sense after that event. While everyone else's world was moving, mine stood still. Life felt numbed out and unreal. When you are 13, life goes by fast. In the first year of my recovery, I missed school dances, band concerts, and lost friends. Grief was there. Sometimes I could not tell whether sadness was related to my illness itself or to the losses I felt. One thing that helped quite a bit was a project from a high school art class. I picked up an old hardcover book and found phrases in it that I related to. I created a collage on each page. At first, I thought of it as just another assignment. But I found looking through pictures and different phrases gave me a way to express certain things. I could find pictures and facial expressions that matched how I was feeling at the moment and had felt at different points. Even after the project was "finished," I kept working on it. I think I worked on it for at least a year.

Mental health conditions are often traumatic. It is normal to feel sad, angry, empty, hurt, and a whole array of other things. It is also typical at times to feel a lack of things—numbness, zoned out, or nothing at all. You might not have words for all of what you are feeling.

You may feel some anger or resentment after developing an illness like this. You might be angry about how others handled your situation or angry that you have to deal with this at all. You may also be struggling to understand why this happened. Sometimes when something bad happens, we look for someone to blame—ourselves or others. With mental health, there is no physical person to blame.

Some also struggle with emotions like embarrassment, guilt, or shame, especially if they had acted in ways they otherwise wouldn't have if not in a mental health episode. It is okay to feel these emotions. It is also important to know that a lot of embarrassment, guilt, and shame related to mental health are unwarranted emotions. You did not ask for this illness. Even if you acted in ways different from how you typically do, those actions were not intentional.

You may also hold some positive emotions. You might feel gratitude for people who were there for you when you were in the worst of your illness. It is also common to have some pride that you made it through. Sometimes, we overlook these emotions in favor of the more negative ones.

Know that whatever you are feeling, your experience is very valid. If you wish to explore your emotions, there are many ways to do this—listening to music you relate to, finding stories with some similarities to your own, through art, fantasy, and conversation. The means of expressing our emotions are almost endless. Everyone has their style.

At first, it may feel overwhelming. You may want to push the emotions away, but this is like trying to hold a beach ball underwater. Just as the beachball pops back up with super force, our emotions often bounce back with energy the more we push away. By allowing yourself to feel these things, you give yourself a chance to feel.

Your Kaleidoscope

What you need

- Some kind of art supply—your choice—colored pencils, crayons, magazine pictures, paints, pens, or just an ordinary pencil.

Take a moment to reflect on the emotions you have felt through this journey. Create an image expressing this. If you have supplies of different colors, feel free to color-code your image. For example, you might choose red for anger or blue for sadness (or maybe you choose blue for anger and red for sadness!). If you wish to draw a pie chart, that is also an option. This is your kaleidoscope!

27

Making Sense of Your Story

Toward the end of high school, a mentor talked to me about a program where I could share my story in classrooms and other places to help other people still struggling. To do that, I had to write down my story first. It took several drafts and some practice, but making sense of my experience and using it to help others sparked a kind of meaning in me.

Taking time to make sense of your story can be an intense but often worthwhile task. When and whether you choose to walk back through your story is a personal choice that only you can make. Still, placing your experiences into words or other expressions can help it make sense. Some people find that in telling their story they feel empowered and more at peace. You might remember the strengths you showed amid this adversity or the people who were there for you.

You may share your story with many people or only one person. Writing it down is one way, but not everyone enjoys writing. Some people process their stories through music, art, talking, or even more creative means. You might make a playlist that describes times in your life or find a specific song that resonates with you. In another direction, you might choose not to try to process your story now, which is also a fine choice.

Therapy can help with this as well.

The exercises that follow will give you a space to process your story with examples of common experiences.

Some people find that they can write a story completely from scratch. If this is you, know that is a talent! Having an outline can help as well. For this reason, we will divide your story into five parts—"before my experience," "during my illness," "getting help," "dealing with my illness now," and "my recovery."

My Story

....

Before my experience

Think back to what you remember before your experience of having a mental health challenge. If you have lived with symptoms for as long as you can remember, think about how things were before your most recent episode. What were you doing? What was important to you?

Example: Before I had a mental health crisis, I loved to play music. I played trumpet in jazz band, concert band, and marching band. I enjoyed philosophy and had a few friends at school.

_____

_____

_____

_____

_____

_____

_____

_____

_____

_____

_____

_____

_____

_____

_____

_____

_____

_____

_____

_____

_____

_____

During my illness

Think about your experiences with your illness, especially before you received help. This is a space to write about symptoms that you may not yet have understood, as well as how people around you reacted. It is okay if emotions come up as you write this. This is normal. If you need a break, feel free to take one.

Example: It started simply enough. I began to enjoy philosophy more. I would spend hours reading and thinking about religion. I stepped away from friends and talked much less. When I did talk, most of what I talked about revolved around religion. I could tell some people around me were freaked out by it. I started thinking about darker topics and feeling depressed. I had no idea I had a mental illness. I did not understand why people were treating me differently. It hurt.

Getting help

You can use this section to process what it was like to get help for your illness. This could include things like going to the hospital, taking medication, talking to a counselor, or joining a first episode psychosis program. Feel free to include both positive and negative pieces.

Example: The day after Easter, my mom took me in the car to a big building with a "buzz-in" type lock. It turned out that that building was a psychiatric hospital. I cried every one of the ten days I was there. I did not think I had a mental illness and was afraid of the medication I was given. I refused it at first, but eventually I tried it. After the hospital, it took time for us to find a good combination of medications that could help me and for me to trust my doctor enough to tell her what was going on. I saw a therapist as well and had group therapy. I liked my therapist even though I did not think I could trust her at first. With time, I started to feel better.

_____

_____

_____

_____

_____

_____

_____

_____

_____

_____

_____

_____

_____

_____

_____

_____

_____

_____

_____

Dealing with my illness

This is a space to write about how you have learned to deal with your illness. You might write about coping skills that you've learned on your own or in therapy as well as how your experience affects your life now.

Example: Dealing with my illness is not always easy. I know now that I need to keep a close eye on triggers, such as how much stress I am under and how much sleep I get. In my first semester in college, I was able to get an accommodation to sign up for classes early so that I could choose all evening classes and sleep in the morning when I struggled with insomnia. I practice strategies like deep breathing and sending well wishes to calm my nerves. I also have found providers I can trust and make sure to attend all of my appointments.

_____

_____

_____

_____

_____

_____

_____

_____

_____

_____

_____

_____

_____

_____

_____

_____

_____

_____

_____

_____

_____

_____

_____

_____

My recovery

In this section, you can share about the accomplishments you have made in your mental health recovery as well as dreams you are pursuing outside mental health. This is a great place to discuss your hopes related to work, school, and relationships.

Example: It has been a while since I have played the trumpet; however, I have found that I enjoy art. I was able to graduate from college and graduate school and now work as a clinical social worker. I love my job. My goals now mostly center around family and having fun in life.

_____

_____

_____

_____

_____

_____

_____

_____

_____

_____

_____

_____

_____

_____

_____

_____

_____

_____

_____

_____

_____

_____

_____

Strategic Disclosure

Knowing Who to Tell and How

I have often wondered about when, with whom, and how I should talk about my illness. It matters to me that people know that I am the same person I always have been. I am still Jen, with or without a diagnosis. I have heard people talk about others with mental illness with unkind phrases such as saying they aren't "all there," or implying that the illness is not real. That is stigma, and I am hesitant to share my own journey with those people. I have found, however, that sharing this part of my life sometimes opens the door for me to relate to others on a level that I would never have otherwise. When I talk about my story, sometimes others tell me about their mental health or another personal connection to it. It is nice to know I am not alone. It is meaningful to consider the pros and cons of sharing your story.

Whether or not to tell someone about your mental health experiences is a personal decision that only you can make. You may decide to tell many people in your life, or you may decide only to tell a few. For example, you may tell your roommate but not every student at your university.

Sharing your story can encourage others to share their own stories or give you an increased sense of support. Unfortunately, sharing your story may also lead to exposure to stigma or stereotypes others have about mental illness. Knowing ahead of time how you might cope if someone responds in less than helpful ways can prepare you for if this does happen.

You can also "test the waters" before deciding whether or not you want to tell someone that you have a mental health condition. You can do this by talking in general about mental health or making known your positive attitudes surrounding mental health. This can give you a sense of whether the people surrounding you will be accepting if you do talk about your challenges.

Lastly, know that how much or little you share is always your choice. If you want to let someone know that you have a mental health condition, that does not mean that you have to tell them about your specific diagnosis or hospitalizations (unless you want to). It is totally up to you how much to share and with whom.

To Share or Not to Share

What are some "pros" of disclosing your illness?

- ☐ Beating stigma
- ☐ Feeling more comfortable
- ☐ Asking for accommodations if I need them
- ☐ Getting closer to someone
- ☐ _____
- ☐ _____

What are some "cons" of disclosing your illness?

- ☐ Stigma
- ☐ Feeling less comfortable
- ☐ I don't like people knowing personal things about me
- ☐ _____
- ☐ _____
- ☐ _____

Who in your life do you feel comfortable talking to about your diagnosis?

1. _____
2. _____
3. _____
4. _____
5. _____

How could you respond if someone reacted in a less than helpful way to your sharing?

- ☐ Seek support from people who understand
- ☐ Provide education about mental health
- ☐ Let the person know that what they said hurt me
- ☐ Leave the conversation
- ☐ _____
- ☐ _____
- ☐ _____

Part 8

CONNECTION

Social Circles

Returning to school after my hospitalization left me feeling like I had missed out on something. I had been in the hospital for two weeks, but it was as if magically an invisible wall was placed between me and everyone else. I did not want people to know about my problems. Still, friendships and support from people like my neighbor, an uncle, and peers in a support group helped me get through those times. Today, relationships are a top priority for me. I have close friends and family in my life.

Relationships are central to most people's lives. These allow us to celebrate the good times, get support in the bad times, and enrich each other's days. Social support is also a big part of many people's recovery. Just having someone to listen and be there for you during points of stress can make it so that you are not facing those things alone.

Right now, you may have strong social circles, such as supportive family members or a teacher you talk to every day. Or you might not. You might find that your social circles are lacking, or that you are having difficulty thinking of anyone you can trust. Wherever you are in terms of your social circles right now, know that growth and change are possible. Taking time to reflect on these circles can help you remember where your strongest supports are as well as the relationships you wish to strengthen.

Social Circles

Take a look at this bullseye.

In the center ring, write the names of people in your closest core group. This could be your closest friends, family members, or important mentors.

In the next ring, write the names of people who are even closer. This could be a friend from your friend group who you hang out with sometimes, or maybe a grandparent.

On the circle closest to the outside, write names of people you know better who you talk to sometimes but not often. This could be someone like a cousin you call every now and then, or a student in your class who says hello sometimes.

On the outside of all the circles, write the names of people you know who theoretically could be supportive to you but who you are not yet close to. This could be someone like a teacher, professor, family member, or peer who you would like to know better. Also write here people you used to be close to but are not currently close to.

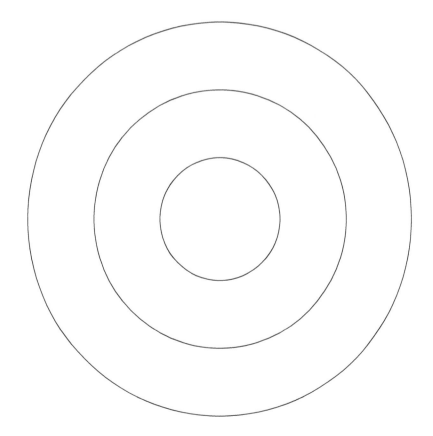

Take another look at your circle. Think about which relationships in your circle you would most like to grow and circle those names. Choose three you most would like to get closer to.

1. _____

2. _____

3. _____

There are many ways to improve a relationship. Some small steps could be:

- ☐ Saying hello
- ☐ Giving a compliment
- ☐ Asking how someone is doing and really listening to what they have to say
- ☐ Looking for a common interest that you have with someone (such as a sports team you both root for)
- ☐ Making a point to say thank you, express gratitude
- ☐ Sending a card or thank-you note
- ☐ Showing body language that signals that you are up to talking (making eye contact, smiling, and letting go of sunglasses or headphones)
- ☐ Doing a random act of kindness
- ☐ Sharing something more personal about yourself
- ☐ Asking someone about something they feel good about (such as a recent accomplishment or interest)
- ☐ Calling someone you have not talked to in a while
- ☐ Sharing a cartoon, news article, or meme that the other person might like
- ☐ Telling a joke
- ☐ Asking for advice
- ☐ Offering to help with something (such as helping a friend move or with a project)
- ☐ _____
- ☐ _____
- ☐ _____

Look back at those three names at the top of this. For each, write one action you could take in the next month to get closer to them.

1. _____

2. _____

3. _____

Building social circles can be hard work. If you do not have many names listed on your social circle above, please do not be discouraged! Sometimes a big part of elevating our social circles is engaging in new communities and meeting new people. Some places you can meet new people are:

- ☐ School
- ☐ Work
- ☐ Exercise clubs (e.g., yoga, a running club)
- ☐ Community centers
- ☐ Volunteering at places (e.g., an animal shelter)
- ☐ Faith communities
- ☐ Organizations at your school (e.g., student council)
- ☐ Organizations in your community (e.g., a charitable organization)

- ☐ _____
- ☐ _____
- ☐ _____

It can take time to get to know people in groups like this, so feel free to start slow. Just a smile or "small talk" conversation can be a good place to start. The next week you might follow up with a deeper question such as "Hey, how did that baseball game you were talking about last week go?" If you don't get the responses you are looking for at first, keep trying! Even talking to one new person is practice for building up supportive circles.

30

Family Support and Triggers

After my hospitalization, I remember hearing family members at a gathering whispering, "I had no idea." They were talking about what had happened to me. It hurt. I wanted to be the one to decide whether to tell them or not. I thought that they would see me as crazy, less trustworthy, and less of a person. Whether that was true or not, I felt treated differently afterwards.

Today, I am more open about my experiences. I recognize that many people struggle with these kinds of things. My family can be supportive to me in my recovery just as they could be in any other challenge. It is important to me that my family knows that I am the same person I was before they knew I had a diagnosis.

Every family is a little different, and we have diverse relationships with our families. For some, family is the strongest of allies. For others, family is a deep source of pain. For many, a family can be both.

Your family could be key in providing support to you in your recovery. At the same time, it is understandable if you have fears surrounding how your family relates to topics regarding your mental health or if you are afraid that your family would treat you differently if they knew about your illness. Stigma attached to mental illness is an unfortunate reality, and families have different understandings of what it means to live with a mental health condition.

Sometimes even when families are doing the best they can, they can still do hurtful things like trying to encourage you "stop being sad" or giving you unwanted advice. In many communities, spaces such as support groups and classes exist to help families care for each other and learn new ways of coping.

For the sake of this workbook, we will use the word "family" broadly to mean the people close to you, not just the people you are biologically related to. The following exercises will explore your relationships with family and what you wish for it.

A Positive Family Memory

Create an image of a positive family memory. Think about what made this memory so good. If you are struggling to think of a positive memory with your biological family, are there people close to you outside your blood family who you could include in your image? If not, create an image of your vision for what you hope to create in your relationships with family.

Reflecting on Family

I need my family to know:

- ☐ That I am the same person I was before my diagnosis
- ☐ That I appreciate them
- ☐ That I am sorry for choices I made during my illness
- ☐ That I am working on my recovery
- ☐ That my illness is treatable
- ☐ That if I forget things more or seem different, these may be symptoms rather than character defects

☐ _____

☐ _____

☐ _____

My family can support me by:

- ☐ Doing the same things together that we did before my illness
- ☐ Learning about mental health recovery
- ☐ Including me in conversations about me
- ☐ Helping me with my return to school and/or work
- ☐ Trusting me to make good choices
- ☐ Attending appointments with me and helping me advocate for myself
- ☐ Helping me keep a clean space
- ☐ Helping me keep a space without bothersome sounds
- ☐ Being willing to repeat themselves sometimes

☐ _____

☐ _____

☐ _____

My family can support me by not:

- ☐ Excluding me from activities
- ☐ Talking about me behind my back
- ☐ Putting pressure on me to _____
- ☐ Making decisions for me without my input

☐ _____

☐ _____

☐ _____

Sometimes even well-meaning family members can do or say things that may trigger our mental health symptoms. Some people also find that being around large groups or noisy spaces such as family gatherings can also be stress triggers.

What is one situation you find triggering with family?

_____

_____

_____

In this situation, what values do you most hope to uphold?
- ☐ To be healthy
- ☐ To be kind
- ☐ To maintain my relationships with family
- ☐ To ask for what I need
- ☐ To say no when I need to
- ☐ To show love
- ☐ To be loved
- ☐ _____
- ☐ _____
- ☐ _____

How can you navigate this situation while still upholding your values?

- ☐ Have a time limit on my family gathering
- ☐ Know that I can leave the family gathering if I need to
- ☐ Have a "safe person" who I can go to if I feel overwhelmed
- ☐ Let one person know about my trigger and how they can support me
- ☐ Make sure I talk to _____ so that even if I have to leave early, I will know I got to visit with this important person
- ☐ Bring _____ with me
- ☐ _____
- ☐ _____
- ☐ _____

31

Communicating With Mental Health Professionals

When I first began receiving mental health treatment, I did not feel my treatment providers were on my side. I did not think that I had a mental illness and believed that the best thing they could do for me would be to leave me alone. I would stop taking my medications a lot. It took a long time before I built trust in a psychiatrist and therapist. One psychiatrist took the time to ask me about college, which I really appreciated as most others just talked to me about my problems. We spent a session talking about that instead of just medications. That was a small part of her showing me that I could trust her. Today, I am thankful for my providers. I believe that they care about my wellbeing and recovery beyond just treating my symptoms. My mental health is extremely important to me. If I cannot keep myself mentally healthy, it is difficult for me to do much else. I know that speaking up for myself in this area and finding supporters I connect with is vital.

Seeking mental health treatment often means encountering several clinicians from different backgrounds. Ultimately, the leader of your treatment is you. These individuals are here to help you in your recovery. Still, you are the best expert on your own experiences, needs, and aspirations. These are some professionals you may meet.

Psychiatrist: A psychiatrist is a medical doctor who specializes in mental health treatment and can prescribe medication and other medical treatments for mental health conditions.

Nurse practitioner: A nurse practitioner is an advanced practice nurse who can also prescribe psychiatric medication.

Recovery support specialist/peer support specialist: A peer recovery support specialist is a person in recovery from a mental health condition or addiction themselves who can offer support, resources, and guidance to others seeking mental health recovery.

Community support specialist: A community support specialist is someone who can help you with resources relating to your independence and recovery goals such as housing, life skills, recreation, community participation, education, work, and other areas. A community support specialist is sometimes also called a key worker or a case worker.

Therapist: A therapist provides psychotherapy to help you move toward your recovery. Therapists come from many backgrounds including marriage/family therapy, counseling, clinical social work, art therapy, psychology, and others.

Vocational rehabilitation specialist: This is someone who can help you with finding and keeping work as well as with your education goals.

If you are experiencing a first episode of psychosis, some communities also offer first episode psychosis coordinated specialty care. This is a fancy term for a team approach within a clinic catered to people who have had an initial psychotic break. If you are unsure if this is available to you, you may reach out to your local community mental health center and ask if they offer a "first episode psychosis program."

While the professionals you see might have years of education, only you know what it is like to be you. If you have questions, ideas, or feelings about your treatment, it is important to make these known.

Some treatment settings offer visual aids such as guides to medication options and their likeliness to cause different side effects. This can help you in these decisions. If you are unsure if this is offered in the clinic you attend, feel free to ask.

What if I disagree with my diagnosis?

Mental health diagnosis is not an exact science, and it is not uncommon for someone to get many different diagnoses, especially when they are first experiencing symptoms. What makes everything more confusing is that, rather than an illness on its own, for most people, psychosis is an overarching symptom. That symptom could have a variety of causes ranging from sleep deprivation to substance use to mental health conditions and other neurological conditions.

You are allowed to disagree with your diagnosis and ask questions! Your perspective matters. In mental health, a person's diagnosis often changes, especially in the early years of someone's illness. What is more important than diagnosis is your goals and aspirations. In your conversations with mental health professionals, try to focus on these as well as any ways that symptoms or medication side effects are affecting your progress toward these things that matter most to you.

Your Mental Health Team

Which mental health professionals are on your team?

- ☐ Psychiatrist
- ☐ Nurse practitioner
- ☐ Community support specialist
- ☐ Peer support specialist
- ☐ Therapist

☐ _____

☐ _____

☐ _____

What would you like the people treating you to know about you (other than your illness)?

_____

_____

_____

_____

_____

What would you like the people treating you to know about your illness?

_____

_____

_____

_____

_____

Getting the Most out of Your Visit With Your Prescriber (Psychiatrist, Nurse Practitioner, etc.)

Preparing topics to discuss with your provider can be helpful to getting the most out of your visit. Feel free to complete this worksheet and bring it with you to your next appointment.

Aspirations that are important to me right now (such as relationship, work, or education goals):

1. _____
2. _____
3. _____

Symptoms that are most affecting my life right now:

1. _____
2. _____
3. _____

Ways medication is helping me:

1. _____
2. _____
3. _____

Side effects I have concerns about:

1. _____
2. _____
3. _____

Other questions I have:

1. _____
2. _____
3. _____

Getting the Most out of Your Visit With Your Therapist

Preparing topics to discuss with your provider can be helpful to getting the most out of your visit. Feel free to complete this worksheet and bring it with you to your next appointment.

Aspirations that are important to me right now (such as relationship, work, or education goals):

1. _____

2. _____

3. _____

Steps I have taken this week toward my aspirations:

1. _____

2. _____

3. _____

Symptoms getting in the way of my aspirations:

1. _____

2. _____

3. _____

Other topics to cover today:

1. _____

2. _____

3. _____

Your Values in Conversation

As a teenager, during my illness, I withdrew a lot. I often did not talk to others and gave off body language meant to send a message that I did not want to talk. I would wear my headphones, look down, and answer questions with one word. As my health improved, I remembered that I like people and wished for better relationships. Rebuilding social circles is hard. It's a "one conversation at a time" kind of thing. When you've kept to yourself for a while, sometimes it is difficult even to think what to talk about. Recognizing what I was aiming to do in a conversation before the actual interaction helped.

Every conversation is a little different. It is helpful to know what your values and goals are in any given interaction. How you interact with someone is likely to vary based on these.

Sometimes our values surround the relationship. We want to get close to the other person, to be present, or have fun. In these situations, it makes sense to show social signals and behaviors that reflect these goals. For example, having a laid-back style, laughter, and being present in the moment reflect these objectives.

Other times, we need to make a request or gather information. In those conversations, it makes sense to be direct and precise. You might have less social chit-chat, although you likely still want to uphold other values you might have about relationships such as being kind and truthful.

Lastly, sometimes your primary goal is to uphold a value. For example, if you wish to fulfill a commitment to another person by helping them with something, acting on your values of loyalty and doing right by that person could be goals in and of themselves.

Whatever your values are, know that you will not hit the target 100 percent of the time. No one does. Still, being intentional and practicing a value of kindness to yourself as you sharpen your skills makes it more likely you will get what you need out of your conversations.

Your Values in Conversation

In most conversations, there is more than one value on the table. For example, you might visit your uncle so that you both can work on a car (completing a task), but you might also want to enjoy your time with your uncle (being present and having fun). Before any major conversation, it can help to take a moment to reflect on what your goal is and what your values are in the conversation.

Some of these could include:

- ☐ Apologizing
- ☐ Asking for something you need
- ☐ Asking a question
- ☐ Being active
- ☐ Being loyal
- ☐ Being kind to others
- ☐ Being present
- ☐ Clarifying instructions
- ☐ Completing a task
- ☐ Confronting someone about a problem
- ☐ Encouraging someone
- ☐ Enjoying time with someone
- ☐ Expressing a worry
- ☐ Figuring out what another person needs
- ☐ Finding a reason to smile
- ☐ Gathering support
- ☐ Getting a need met
- ☐ Getting closer to someone
- ☐ Giving support
- ☐ Having fun
- ☐ Helping someone with something
- ☐ Keeping a commitment to someone
- ☐ Learning something new from someone
- ☐ Making someone laugh
- ☐ Making someone smile
- ☐ Protecting yourself or someone you love
- ☐ Showing appreciation

☐ Sharing something important to you
☐ Standing up for your values
☐ Telling the truth

☐ _____

☐ _____

☐ _____

Keeping the value you have in mind before you enter any conversation is super helpful. Your valued goals are likely to change in different situations, and so how you go about things will show that. If your main goal is to get a need met, you will likely approach the conversation differently than if you are wishing to just get to know someone better.

Think of an upcoming interaction. What is one value that you hope to act on?

_____

If your values include getting closer to someone, it can also help to think of conversation topics ahead of time.

Who is one person you would like to get to know better?

_____

What are three questions that might help you get to know this person better?

1. _____

2. _____

3. _____

Asking for What You Need

I feel like teenagers aren't taught how to stand up for themselves. When I was a teen, I wasn't. I was told to listen to the people around me who knew better than I did. But being able to speak up and to ask for things is so important. A good part of life is a series of negotiations. I've put a lot of practice into this.

Every person's experience is unique. Still, assertiveness is not a commonly taught skill. Even when young people speak up, many report not feeling that they are taken seriously. Young people are routinely not given much voice in decisions that affect them. If you find yourself struggling with how to ask for what you need, know that you are not alone.

Some people struggle to speak up. Other people are taught or modeled ways of asserting themselves that are less effective, such as yelling to be heard or using power plays. Finally, some people are taught effective ways to ask about their needs. If this is you, that's great!

Wherever you are on this continuum, learning to ask for what you need and expressing what matters to you are valuable skills.

We can practice asking for what we need and living our values in formal and informal settings. The two sometimes look a little different, though.

Here are some tips for asking for what you need in a formal setting such as at a pharmacy or the financial aid department at a college:

Be kind: Most people do want to help. While it can be tempting to give some-one a hard time or use sarcasm in frustrating situations, it rarely helps. You may also have a general value of treating others with kindness.

Write down your questions ahead of time: Remembering questions on the spot is challenging. Writing down your question will help you make sure everything you wish to be covered is covered.

Prioritize what you want to talk about: There may be several topics you wish to talk about in certain settings. Write these down and rank them according to what is most important to you.

Assume the best: Sometimes things are unclear. For example, if someone does not call you back, it may be tempting to assume that they don't like you. Still, no one can read minds. It is at least as likely that the person may have called the wrong number, forgotten, or something else. It generally does us well to assume the best.

Follow up: If you are advocating for yourself in a formal setting, you might not get all of your questions answered on the same day. Schedule a time to follow up. This could be as simple as saying, "If I don't hear back from you by Wednesday next week, I will follow up with an email."

Show gratitude: When you are asking for someone's assistance, it is always helpful to show gratitude. You can do this by thanking the person, expressing appreciation, or even sending a card if the situation calls for it.

In informal settings, there may also be times that you speak up for yourself. Many of the above strategies can be helpful, especially showing gratitude or assuming the best. However, in less formal spaces you may also use these tips:

Signal appreciation: A simple thing such as saying "thank you" or "I appreciate you" can go a long way. Other ways to signal appreciation in an informal setting include showing social signals that indicate care and humility. Social signals such as putting away electronics when with someone or listening to what someone has to say can go a long way.

Give back: Meaningful relationships are usually a two-way street. We give help/assistance at times and receive it at other times.

Asking for something

Asking for something can be intimidating. What follows is a simple way to do this: **LAND.**

First, you need to figure out what you want to ask for. Know beforehand as best as you can.

This is what LAND stands for:

L: Let the person know what's up

Let the person know about the situation first with just the facts and then how it is impacting you.

Example: I saw your truck parked in front of my driveway. It is making it difficult to get my vehicle out of the lot.

A: Ask for what you need

Ask for what you need. Be specific.

Example: Would you be up to parking your truck a few feet past my driveway?

N: Negotiate as needed

Sometimes a person does what you ask right off the bat and there is no need to negotiate. Still, more often than not, some degree of negotiation happens.

Example: (Say the person you are talking to lets you know that there is not enough room to park past your driveway. You might be able to come to a shared solution.) There are places to park on the next street.

D: Do it in a way that shows your values

However you ask, do it in a way that shows the values that are important to you. These could include any of the values listed on the previous pages as well as things like honesty, kindness, self-respect, and getting a need met.

Example: (If you value kindness, you might practice strategies of assuming the best, using language that is courteous, and trying to work with the other person. You can practice these by keeping an open posture and taking time to listen to the other person while also asserting your own needs.) Parking around here is often tricky; I hope you can find a suitable space.

Negotiating Your Needs

Think about something you'd like to ask for and complete the following exercise to practice LAND.

What are you asking for? (Be specific)

_____

_____

L: Let the person know what's up

_____

_____

A: Ask for what you need

_____

_____

N: Negotiate as needed

What problems might the other person bring up? What negotiations are you willing to make?

_____

_____

D: Do it in a way that shows your values

What values matter to you in this conversation?

_____

_____

How can you do this in a way that shows your values?

_____

_____

Standing up for Yourself

"Boundaries" has become a sort of buzzword recently. I think it is great that we are finally talking about this. Still, I don't know that everyone means the same thing when they say "boundaries." For me, setting boundaries is setting a line between myself and others that keeps me safe but is not so rigid as to block me from my valued goals. For example, setting my boundaries might mean saying how late I am prepared to stay out or what I am comfortable with in different situations. I used to think setting boundaries meant giving less of myself, but that is not true. It's letting people know what I need and where I stand with my values so that I can live my life how I wish.

There are a lot of misunderstandings surrounding things like "assertiveness," "boundaries," and speaking up, so let's talk about these first.

- ✗ **Myth:** "Assertiveness is another word for learning to be mean."
- ✓ **Fact:** Most people appreciate direct communication. Think of it this way: If a close friend of yours was not okay with something, would you want them to tell you or hide it? Direct communication is a sign of respect.

- ✗ **Myth:** "Boundaries are rules."
- ✓ **Fact:** Boundaries represent your social values and personal needs. These are not meant to be punitive. People only know your boundaries if you communicate them.

- ✗ **Myth:** "If someone crosses your boundaries, you should cut them off."
- ✓ **Fact:** There are situations where someone repeatedly crosses boundaries, and leaving the relationship is the best choice we can make for our health. Still, boundary crossings happen every day. There is a whole rainbow of strategies that you can use to make your boundaries known when needed. Healthy relationships often involve patterns of conflict and resolution.

- ✗ **Myth:** "You don't get to be assertive or have boundaries until you are an adult."

✓ **Fact:** Standing up for ourselves and making our values and needs known is something we can practice throughout our lives.

✗ **Myth:** "Some people are naturally assertive and other people aren't."
✓ **Fact:** Effective communication is a skill anyone can develop. Still, assertiveness might be different from person to person.

Boundaries

Boundaries demark how we want to live our lives in terms of our values as well as what we are okay with (and not okay with) in our relationships. We have boundaries in a variety of areas such as:

- health (e.g., a boundary of giving yourself eight hours to sleep no matter what)
- relationships (e.g., a boundary of valuing truth and wishing to be told the truth)
- safety (e.g., a boundary of not riding in the car with an intoxicated person)
- time (e.g., how many hours a week you are available to work)
- property (e.g., whether you are okay with letting someone drive your car)
- values (e.g., you may not be okay with lying on someone else's behalf).

These are just a small number of areas that we have boundaries in; however, you may think of others personal to you. We can set boundaries in virtually any area of our lives.

There are three types of boundaries:

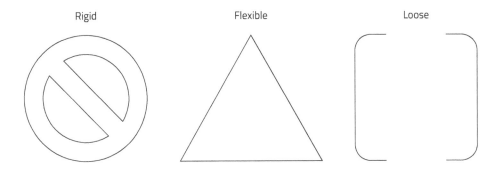

| Rigid | Flexible | Loose |

Most of us have different styles of boundaries for different situations. It is okay to change your boundaries when you need to. All of these boundaries can also be healthy in the right situations.

Rigid boundaries

These are boundaries that are solid and unchanging, and which you are not easily talked out of. Most people have at least a few rigid boundaries—for example, involving health and safety issues. They are sort of like a prohibition or stop sign.

Flexible boundaries

These are boundaries that are important but can also be changed depending on the situation. You can think of them like a caution sign, flexible enough to change as needed but clear enough for others to know your boundary. For example, you might have a flexible boundary surrounding how much time you spend practicing an instrument. Under normal circumstances, maybe you spend no more than a few hours practicing each week, but you are willing to practice more before a big concert.

Loose boundaries

These are low-priority boundaries that are more like preferences. For example, some people prefer their friends to ask before grabbing a soda from their cooler, but if a friend doesn't ask, they won't get too hung up about it

Your Boundaries in Different Life Spaces

What are some of your boundaries...

In terms of health?

_____

_____

_____

In your relationships?

_____

_____

_____

With safety?

_____

_____

_____

For your time?

_____

_____

_____

For your property?

_____

_____

_____

Your Boundary Levels

What is one rigid boundary that you have?

_____

_____

_____

What is one loose boundary that you have?

_____

_____

_____

What is one flexible boundary that you have?

_____

_____

_____

Are there boundaries you currently have that you would like to make more flexible?

_____

_____

_____

_____

_____

What would that look like?

_____

_____

_____

_____

_____

Part 9

YOUR RECOVERY

Getting Moving Again

For a long time, I felt frozen. When you are 13, life moves fast. At age 13, between Easter and the second week of the following school year, I had three hospitalizations. I sort of started "hiding out." I didn't leave my room much, missed a lot of school, and didn't really have friends. Looking at my life was like looking at a forest that had been mostly destroyed. I felt left behind. I did not know how to get moving again and it felt like doing so would take longer than I was able to cope with. But what I learned was I didn't have to re-forest the forest right away. Doing little things like going to the library, taking a walk, or calling someone I had been avoiding helped me slowly reclaim the things that are important to me.

A mental health crisis is a life-changing event. If you are having trouble getting moving again after yours, know that you are not alone. There are many things that may have changed since your illness like friendships, how you feel, what activities you participate in, and changes to school or work. As time has gone by, you may have also gone through other changes, such as a move, or you may have seen changes in the lives of the people around you.

It might be hard to remember what you value or imagine mapping a way forward. The good news is that it does not have to happen all at once. Think about what has mattered to you in the past. How do you want to be remembered? When do you feel at your best? Then dial back from there. What is one small step you can take in that direction?

It is possible to take steps toward the things that are important to us every day. If friendship is important to you, a small step could be sending a meme to someone you used to talk to or making a point to smile at someone. If you used to enjoy having fun, a small step could be visiting an arcade or flying a kite. Just keep moving bit by bit toward what matters to you.

Your Dreams and Your Values

If you knew you had one year left to live, what are three things that you would want to do?

1. _____

2. _____

3. _____

What does this tell you about what is important to you?

_____

_____

_____

_____

Something neat is that we can take steps toward our values, the things that really matter to us, each day. Check out this list of common values and small steps you can take. Feel free to add your own. Check off steps you would be open to taking.

Achievement

- ☐ Write a list of goals
- ☐ Do one small thing on my to-do list
- ☐ Do a small chore
- ☐ Fill out a college or job application
- ☐ Choose a skill I would like to learn and watch a video about it
- ☐ Practice a skill I would like to learn such as writing or skateboarding for 15 minutes

- ☐ _____
- ☐ _____
- ☐ _____

Adventure

- ☐ Go to a place I have never been
- ☐ Explore a park
- ☐ Attend a group or club at school or a library
- ☐ Visit a community center

☐ Explore my neighborhood

☐ _____

☐ _____

☐ _____

Connection

☐ Call an old friend
☐ Write a letter to someone
☐ Thank someone
☐ Smile at someone
☐ Ask someone a question about themselves

☐ _____

☐ _____

☐ _____

Creativity

☐ Listen to a song I have never heard before
☐ Doodle
☐ Make up my own recipe
☐ Write a poem
☐ Do something unexpected

☐ _____

☐ _____

☐ _____

Gratitude

☐ Write a list of good things
☐ Write a thank-you letter to someone who has helped me
☐ Tell someone something I appreciate about them

☐ _____

☐ _____

☐ _____

Helping others

- ☐ Ask for an application to volunteer for a cause important to me
- ☐ Bake or cook a dish that I know someone in my home loves
- ☐ Help a family member, friend, or neighbor with yard work or a chore
- ☐ Offer to listen to someone needing someone to talk to
- ☐ Share an uplifting story, quote, or meme
- ☐ Take a pet for a walk

- ☐ _____
- ☐ _____
- ☐ _____

Learning new things

- ☐ Pick something that I have always wanted to learn about and do an internet search
- ☐ Visit a library
- ☐ Ask someone about something they know about
- ☐ Read
- ☐ Sign up for a class
- ☐ Choose a skill I would like to learn

- ☐ _____
- ☐ _____
- ☐ _____

Nature

- ☐ Look at a leaf up close
- ☐ Listen to the birds
- ☐ Visit a park
- ☐ Help clean a space in my neighborhood
- ☐ Practice stargazing
- ☐ Appreciate a sunset or sunrise

- ☐ _____
- ☐ _____
- ☐ _____

Self-acceptance

- ☐ Share something about myself with another person
- ☐ Practice expressing myself with my appearance
- ☐ Journaling

- ☐ _____
- ☐ _____
- ☐ _____

What other values do you have? What steps could you take toward those values?

_____
_____
_____
_____

Consider some things you checked off in the last exercise. On the following page, you will find a planner for which to engage these values in real life. Write some down that you may be able to do in the next week. The goal of this exercise is to practice planning. If you don't do everything you write, that's okay! However, each activity you do is a step toward getting moving again.

	Monday	Tuesday	Wednesday	Thursday	Friday	Saturday	Sunday
8am–10am							
10am–12pm							
12pm–2pm							
2pm–4pm							
4pm–6pm							
6pm–8pm							
8pm–10pm							

36

School

After my final hospitalization, I missed 30 days of school. I was supposed to do home-schooling, but that didn't happen. After so long, a meeting took place at my school. I was given a chance to go to a therapeutic school for students living with mental health challenges. At first, I did not want to go. I thought that schools like this were for "bad" or "crazy" kids and that attending there would hold me back from my dreams. But I gave it a shot. It was hard at first, and I did miss a lot of school. Still, within six months, I had a friend, and within a year, my grades had risen from not passing to mostly As. I could do this.

Mental health symptoms have a way of interrupting our plans. You may have missed school due to mental health symptoms or time spent in treatment, especially hospital. In addition, it is hard to concentrate and do your best at school when coping with significant mental health symptoms.

Returning to school after a mental health crisis tends to bring both hopes and fears. You may have fears about things such as managing symptoms at school. Still, you likely also have some hopes about school such as being able to graduate or return to a club you used to enjoy. Many people can successfully return to school after a mental health crisis.

Everyone has their own pace for returning to school. If you do not feel ready to go back to school for an entire day, you may wish to ask if returning to school for half days is an option until you find yourself healthy enough to get through the whole day. Some school districts also offer alternative programming or evening classes with fewer people, which some may find less overwhelming.

Your school may offer you accommodations for your experience. This could be assistance, such as being able to leave class to visit the school counselor during times you feel overwhelmed. It could also be adjustments like having a seat near the front of the classroom if you find yourself distracted by things in front of you (or in the back of the classroom if that is what you are most comfortable with). Some students also receive services at school or accommodations through special arrangements.

The person who knows best what you need is you. Speaking up to express concerns or asking for specific accommodations are things you can do to get what you need. You can write down what difficulties, concerns, and goals you have as you return to school, and any ideas you have about how the school can support you can give your team a blueprint.

Reaching out to a mentor can also be helpful. This could be a peer counselor through a local mental health agency, another student, a person working in a field you currently work in, or a person working in a field you would like to work in. A mentor can encourage you and help you to stay on track.

Your Hopes and Fears for School

As you think about returning to school, what are your top three hopes?

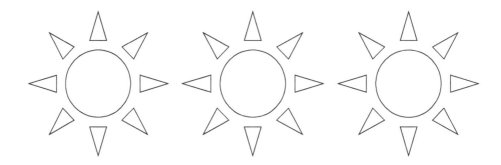

What are your top three fears about returning to work, school, or volunteering?

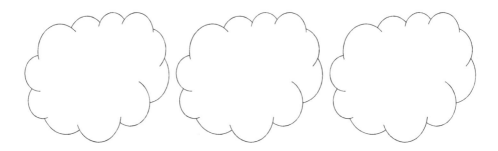

Often we find that as we get closer to our hopes, we also find our anxieties rising. Returning to work, school, or volunteering after a mental health crisis is a major change. Still, it can be extremely meaningful.

What would be the best part about returning to school?

_____

_____

_____

_____

_____

_____

Your Concerns About School

Conversations with key people at school can be difficult. Having a list of your concerns, goals, and ideas for what might help can make it easier.

Check off any of these common school-related concerns which you identify with.

- ☐ Difficulties concentrating
- ☐ Crowds
- ☐ Past bad experiences at school
- ☐ Anxiety about going to school
- ☐ Stress related to large projects
- ☐ Working with other people in group projects
- ☐ Keeping up with homework
- ☐ Bullying at school
- ☐ Catching up after having missed school
- ☐ Noise
- ☐ Depression making it difficult to go to school
- ☐ Difficulty waking in time for school
- ☐ Hallucinations at school
- ☐ Feeling like people are staring at me
- ☐ Feeling like people are talking about me
- ☐ Feeling like someone has it in for me

Addressing Your School-Related Concerns

While these are complex challenges, there are certain things you might find helpful. Some of these are accommodations the school could put in place to help you; others are things that you might be able to do on your own. Here are some ideas for each concern from the previous activity; check those which you think could be helpful to you.

Difficulties concentrating

☐ Ask a teacher or classmate for copies of notes
☐ Practice re-focusing on bringing my mind back over and over to class
☐ Take a short break if allowed

Crowds

☐ An accommodation to transition between classes 5–10 minutes early
☐ An accommodation of a smaller class
☐ Practice breathing exercises as I walk through the halls
☐ Practice positive self-talk or a mantra during transition periods

Past bad experiences at school

☐ Talk with my school social worker or a counselor about my experience
☐ Write my experience down
☐ Focus on creating new positive school memories
☐ Process my prior bad school experiences with a therapist

Anxiety about going to school

☐ An accommodation of beginning with half days
☐ Setting my things out the night before
☐ Reviewing my plan for the next day the night before
☐ De-catastrophizing—reminding myself that my mind can tell me many stories about bad things that could happen but that my mind has told me many stories in the past of things that never happened

Stress related to large projects

☐ Breaking my projects down into smaller pieces
☐ Writing down all large projects at the beginning of the semester in an agenda book and then break them into steps

Working with other people in group projects

- ☐ Ask for an accommodation of choosing my groups for group projects
- ☐ Use a specific notebook for my group project and write the overall goal in one color and my part in another color

Keeping up with homework

- ☐ Keep an agenda book
- ☐ Make a space in my home my study space with everything I need to study
- ☐ Set aside a space outside my home to study and do homework (e.g., a library)
- ☐ Do homework at the same time every day
- ☐ Listen to music while doing homework if it helps me concentrate
- ☐ Have a special treat only while I do homework (e.g., gummy worms)

Bullying at school

- ☐ Power in numbers—staying near one or two good friends
- ☐ Talking to someone at my school about my experience
- ☐ Join anti-bullying clubs at my school

Catching up after having missed school

- ☐ Create a plan with my school social worker and teachers to help me catch up
- ☐ Divide all I need to do into small parts and do a little each day
- ☐ Ask for an accommodation of extended time to complete my assignments

Noise

- ☐ Ask for an accommodation of noise-canceling headphones
- ☐ Practice mindfulness strategy of focusing on my breath
- ☐ Sit in an area of the classroom that is less loud (such as in the front)

Depression making it difficult to go to school

- ☐ Ask for an accommodation of a half day or beginning school later
- ☐ Remember my reasons for wanting to finish school
- ☐ Talk to my psychiatrist and therapist about my depression
- ☐ Celebrate days I am able to go to school
- ☐ Be kind to myself
- ☐ Remember it is not all or nothing—doing some school work is better than none

Difficulty waking in time for school

- ☐ Ask for an accommodation of a half day or beginning school later or night classes
- ☐ Ask for an accommodation of beginning my school day with an active class like gym
- ☐ Use an alarm with music I like
- ☐ Set my alarm far away from my bed so that it is difficult to turn off

Hallucinations at school

- ☐ Ask for an accommodation of being able to leave class if I am experiencing an hallucination
- ☐ Ask for an accommodation to bring headphones to school for days when my voices are loud
- ☐ Bring something to school that I can fidget with to help me re-focus and cope
- ☐ Practice a positive mantra for coping with hallucinations
- ☐ Talk with my psychiatrist or therapist about how this symptom affects me

Feeling like people are staring at me

- ☐ Ask for an accommodation of seating in the front or back row
- ☐ Put it into perspective: If people are staring at me, what is the worst that can happen? Will I survive? Will I remember this in five years?

Feeling like people are talking about me at school

- ☐ Ask for an accommodation of seating in the front or back row
- ☐ Put it into perspective: If people are staring at me, what is the worst that can happen? Will I survive? Will I remember this in five years?

Feeling like someone has it in for me

- ☐ Power in numbers: Find one or two people at my school whom I can trust
- ☐ Put it into perspective: Ask myself what makes me believe that someone has it in for me? Is there evidence against this thought? Are there other possible explanations?

37

Work or Volunteering

My first "job" after my mental health crisis (which also happened to be my first job ever) was volunteering at a summer camp. I liked that I got to help people, I got to work with kids, it was incredibly fun, and it was time-limited. Becoming a summer camp counselor was not my end-goal job, but it was a huge step for me. I learned a lot, met some cool people, and worked at summer camps for the next three years.

Returning to or beginning work after a mental health crisis can be intimidating. Many people re-enter the workplace part-time or start with volunteer opportunities. If you have never worked, discovering what kind of work you might enjoy will be the first step to entering the workforce. Similarly, if you have worked or are working, it may also be worthwhile to determine if the work you do still aligns with your strengths, values, and needs at this time. These are big questions.

In most communities, resources exist to help you sort through your work-related needs, strengths, and interests. Resources such as job centers, or what is known as "vocational rehabilitation," are career development services catering to people who have disabilities that can be of support. Programs such as this may offer services to help you find job opportunities, practice interview skills, provide mentorship, and sometimes even assist with the costs of college or job training.

You may be eligible for accommodations at work. Requesting accommodations could require you to disclose your status as a person with a need for accommodation, which has pros and cons. Still, accommodations can help ensure your success. Assistance could include adaptations like having a morning shift if your medication makes you less productive in the evening, allowance for time off work to attend therapy and psychiatric appointments, or working from home during high symptom days.

Sharing your mental health challenges in the workplace can bring up a lot of fears. You might worry that you would lose your job or lose opportunities if other people knew about your challenges. While not everyone has a mental health condition, everyone has mental health. Many workplaces have some experience or resources surrounding mental health. Still, stigma is real, and, unfortunately, some people experience negative consequences when they share their experiences. It is perfectly okay if you do not want to disclose your diagnosis. You get to decide who you wish to disclose to and how much you want to share.

Volunteering is also an excellent place to try out different jobs, build job skills, and build connections to help you if you choose paid employment. Some benefits of volunteering include:

- a chance to help others
- a setting that is often more flexible than traditional employment
- a space where you can try out multiple different roles
- a chance to practice job skills
- opportunities to build connections which could help you to find work.

Your Dream Job

Let's take a minute to dream. What is your dream job? If you struggle to think of something right off the bat, see if you can relate to something that you may have wanted to do in the past. What makes that job sound or feel like such a good fit? What would be the best part of working at this particular job?

_____

_____

_____

_____

_____

_____

_____

Most times we are attracted to work that:

- is interesting to us
- we could imagine ourselves enjoying
- is based on something we are good at
- aligns with our values.

Most of us do not begin work with our "dream job," and what we consider our "dream job" could change over time. For example, to become a veterinarian you would need to first complete the necessary schooling. If you do not yet have that schooling, work as a veterinary assistant, as a teammate at a kennel, or at a humane society could help you to build up those skills until you have the schooling you need.

If you cannot start with your dream job, what jobs can you think of which have some similarities to your dream job?

_____

_____

_____

_____

_____

_____

_____

Volveteering

Volunteering can be a bridge to paid employment and has many advantages in its own right. Your community likely has several spaces that accept volunteers. Look at the list of popular venues for volunteering and check off any you'd be interested to find out more about.

- ☐ Animal shelters
- ☐ Nursing homes
- ☐ Summer camps
- ☐ Senior centers
- ☐ Youth programs
- ☐ Programs that serve individuals with disabilities (such as Special Olympics or beauty pageants just for people living with a disability)
- ☐ Food banks
- ☐ Mental health organizations
- ☐ Mentorship programs
- ☐ Shelters for the unhoused
- ☐ Thrift stores

- ☐ Libraries
- ☐ Community fitness centers
- ☐ Disaster relief organizations
- ☐ Parks
- ☐ Churches
- ☐ Museums
- ☐ Advocacy groups for specific causes (e.g., fighting cancer or world hunger)
- ☐ Adult education programs
- ☐ _____
- ☐ _____
- ☐ _____

You can also consider what tasks you most would be interested in doing. For example, if you enjoy writing, you may ask about an organization's newsletter. If working directly with people is more your thing or if this is something you would like to develop, you might ask about opportunities to volunteer providing direct service, such as working directly with the residents at a local nursing care center. There also is often a high need for help with other tasks such as sorting mail or goods (like the food at a food pantry).

Some mental health organizations also welcome volunteers to share their stories of living with a mental health condition or to assist with educational programs. Everyone's story is unique, and by sharing our stories we can help to create change. Many find this to be especially meaningful.

When thinking about volunteering, are there any causes or spaces which come to mind as doing work that is important to you or that you would be interested in joining in?

_____

_____

_____

_____

38

What Are Your Hopes and Dreams?

Before my illness, I wanted to be a music teacher. That continued to be my main dream through the start of high school, but I found that what I used to enjoy—playing the trumpet and writing music—no longer gave me joy. So, I stopped doing those things. My interest faded, especially after I started at a school with no band.

I still think if I wanted to, I could have pursued that. But my new school had a different opportunity for me—a peer-to-peer mentoring deal. I signed up for that and learned that encouraging others is something I love. I created a new hope—to be a therapist. I also focused on day-to-day things like trying to speak up more at school to get to know people and make friends. Going to college was also a dream of mine. Preparing for that involved several steps—taking the ACT, searching for schools that could be a good fit for me, and applying to college. But it happened. I finished college, finished graduate school, and became a therapist.

When we are struggling with our mental health, often the focus is on making bad things—like mental health symptoms—go away. Mental health symptoms can temporarily eclipse our goals and dreams. While managing symptoms is meaningful, there is much more to life. Recovery is about creating and moving toward hopes and dreams.

Our lives have multiple dimensions, and recovery usually involves targets within each of these.

Some areas of life goals include:

- having fun
- education goals
- social goals
- work goals
- financial/asset-type goals
- health goals.

Recovery goals can be specific—like finishing a class—but can also relate to less tangible things like having fun. Beginning a new hobby or attending a

Dungeons and Dragons club each week could totally be part of a recovery vision. Similarly, health is something most people value, and so you may have dreams surrounding your health, such as a goal of learning how to swim.

When considering dreams, don't hold back. If you don't believe that a dream is realistic right now, that's okay. We will talk about breaking up big dreams into smaller steps in the next section. The important thing is seeking out visions that energize and inspire you.

It is essential to make sure that whatever dreams you choose are, in fact, your dreams. Not your parents', not your doctors', but visions that matter to you. You might ask others for ideas, but at the end of the day, this is your life and your recovery.

Finally, it is perfectly normal for your dreams to change with time. Some of your hopes today may be the same dreams you have five years from now. Others you could decide to move on from in time. When creating recovery visions, it is helpful to be open and flexible.

Your Dreams

What would be your dreams? Don't hold back or question if they are realistic or not. This is a chance for you to draw up a vision. Consider the following areas of your life.

Having fun (such as places you'd like to go or things you'd like to do):

_____

_____

_____

Education (such as something you'd like to learn more about, higher education goals, or job training goals):

_____

_____

_____

Social (such as friendship or romantic goals):

_____

_____

_____

Work (such as what kind of job you might like):

_____

_____

_____

Assets (such as getting a driver's license, saving money, or opening a bank account):

_____

_____

_____

Health (such as feeling more energy or getting stronger):

_____

_____

_____

Choose one of these areas and draw yourself living your dream in this box.

Your Dreams for the Next Year

For each of these visions, write a goal that you might be able to accomplish in the next year. This is a long-term goal.

Having fun (Example: Go fishing once a month):

_____

_____

_____

Education (Example: Apply to three colleges):

_____

_____

_____

Social (Example: Improve my friendship with Juan):

_____

_____

_____

Work (Example: Find a job):

_____

_____

_____

Assets (Example: Get my driver's license):

_____

_____

_____

Health (Example: Go to the gym once a week every week):

_____

_____

_____

Taking Steps Toward Your Dreams

Choosing a dream of becoming a mental health professional gave me hope. In high school, that dream felt so far away. Most of the jobs I wished for required a college degree and some days just getting through the school day overwhelmed me. One thing that encouraged me was doing small things that moved me toward my dream and keeping sight of the reasons it mattered to me. I used my class projects to learn about topics related to my interests, took a mental health recovery class at a local church, and worked toward finishing my diploma. Sometimes my step for the day was getting up and going to school.

Moving toward bigger goals will almost always take a series of small steps. Some of the steps will lead directly toward the goal—for example, finishing a paper so that you can pass a class. Others might be less obvious such as going to a community event to reaccustom yourself to being around people again as you work toward a goal of returning to work. Both are important.

It's easy to get caught up in goals, and, of course, goals matter. Still, achieving a goal is a small piece of time compared to all the time we spend working toward that goal. Each step matters too. And what is even more vital is the reason behind the goal—why you want to accomplish it in the first place, and your values.

Rather than thinking only of your greater vision, it can be helpful to think about *why* this matters to you and to start there. From there, you can look for small things that you can do each day not only to inch toward your goal but also to live your values. You don't have to wait until you reach your goal to have the satisfaction of living a life rooted in your values.

In the same vein, each step is an opportunity to celebrate. In Dialectical Behavioral Therapy (DBT), this is called "building mastery." Completing even one step or mastering a new activity is a win.

Stepping Stones Toward a Dream

Think of a larger goal you have, such as one you may have identified in the previous chapter.

Write it here.

_____

_____

_____

On the stepping stones below, write steps you can take toward your larger goal. Once you have a list, feel free to write a number on each in order of which steps to do first, second, third. If you cannot place these in an order or are not able to do the steps in the order you first imagine, that is okay! Each step is a step forward.

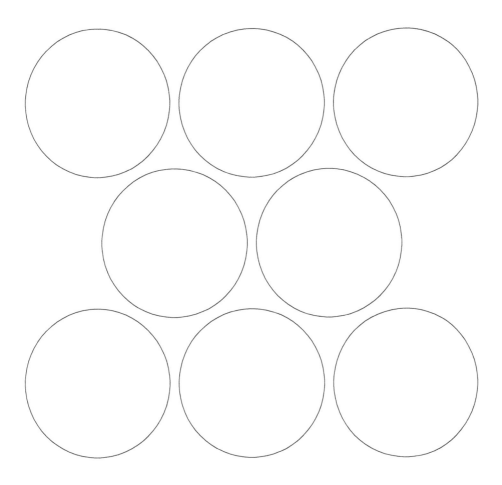

Celebrating the Good Things

What ways can you celebrate as you check off each step?

- ☐ Remembering why this matters to me
- ☐ Doing something fun
- ☐ Telling someone close to me
- ☐ Writing my success in a journal or on social media
- ☐ Enjoying a snack
- ☐ Checking it off a list

- ☐ _____
- ☐ _____
- ☐ _____

Keeping up Your Garden

Maintaining Your Recovery

While sometimes I wished my mental health story ended with a full recovery around age 14, happily ever after and all, the reality is my recovery has been and will be an everyday thing. Each day, I take part in activities to maintain my health—both physical and mental. At times, I encounter triggers. I use tools every day to maintain my wellness and am constantly sharpening my tools. Sometimes I find a need for new tools too! I have grown in compassion for myself and others along the way. I hope that I never stop learning. There is so much in life to discover and experience.

Some things we only do once. Graduating high school is typically a one-time thing. You do the work, pass the classes, walk across the stage (or don't), and you're done. Other things have to be maintained.

Think of a garden full of vibrant flowers. Each of those flowers is a living being with changing needs. For the garden to thrive, someone will need to keep up with the garden by watering plants, pulling weeds, and sometimes throwing down new seeds. In the same way, upholding mental health is an ongoing ride.

Like a gardener watering their plants, we also need to do things that keep us healthy. This could be things like spending time with people who encourage us, or attending appointments with treatment team members. We also need to have "just enough" of certain things. Sleeping too little or too much could both lead to difficulties in the right circumstances.

Just as weeds come up in a garden, triggers for mental health symptoms are bound to pop up in all of our lives. These difficulties could be a conflict with a close friend, stress, a loss, or any number of life changes. We need to tend to ourselves in the face of these triggers, and these triggers could also mean a change in needs.

Lastly, just as the gardener throws down new seeds, we need to give ourselves space and means to grow. Moving toward goals, fostering treasured relationships, or engaging in fun and meaningful activities are ways to grow. As life changes, our needs and passions often do too.

Recovery is a forever thing. And that's okay. Continuous growth brings color and meaning to life.

Watering Your Garden

Think of your "garden." What are some things you can do to water your garden or help you stay healthy? Write these on the water drops:

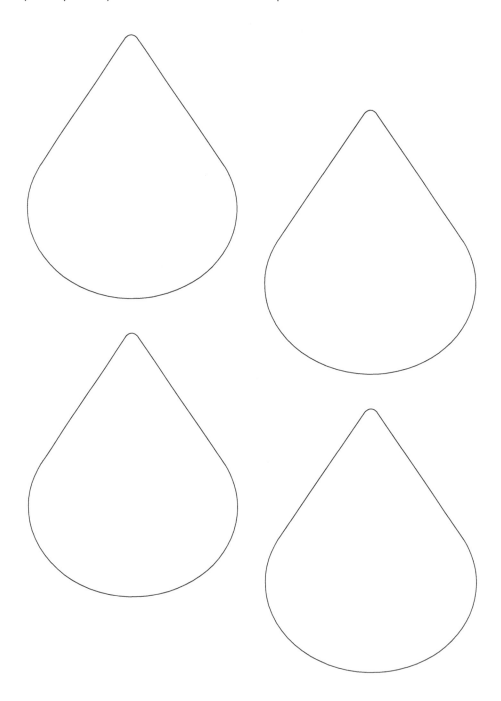

Dealing With Storms

Now, think of some possible triggers that could affect your recovery. Write these on the lightning bolts. Alongside each lightning bolt, write your plan for that trigger.

Plan

Plan

Planting Seeds

Lastly, think of areas for growth and ways you can keep growing. Write one of these on each of the seeds below.

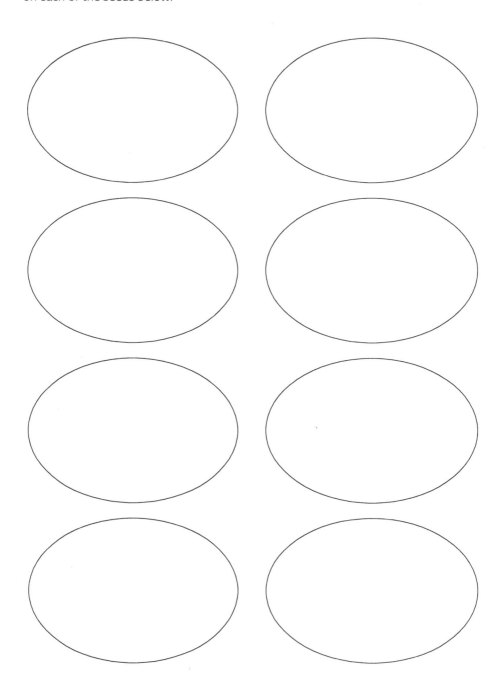

Part 10

THE BIGGER PICTURE

Fighting Stigma

Before I knew I had mental health conditions myself, I did not know much about mental illness. I knew about anxiety, but I thought somewhere in the mist there were also "crazy people" out there—hiding out in asylums, totally out of touch. When I was first hospitalized and given a diagnosis, I wondered if I was a "crazy person." I thought that others would not see me as a whole person—that they would think that I wasn't "all there." Over the years that followed, my whole perspective changed. I don't believe anyone is "crazy." Those pictures in my mind that I had of "crazy people" could not be farther from the truth of people I have met living with mental health conditions. Everyone has mental health and, just as we can struggle with our physical health, some of us also struggle with our mental health.

Today I know that living with a mental health condition is not a choice any more than having epilepsy or heart disease is. It doesn't make you weak to live with these kinds of things. Seeking treatment and recovery takes strength. I have a lot of respect for anyone who lives with mental health conditions. I fight stigma by sharing my story with those close to me and educating others when I encounter myths about mental illness. As a society, we have come a long way, but we still have a way to go in terms of understanding mental health and creating a world that is friendly to individuals struggling with mental health.

Stigma is a kind of negative social notion that paints a picture of people with mental health conditions that is not accurate. This often includes false ideas such as that mental illness is all "in your head" or that people with mental health conditions are dangerous. Stigma discourages people from getting help and makes it harder for people with mental health conditions to be their best.

Let's face it, stigma sucks. But there are some things we can do about it.

Many schools and communities have dedicated clubs, organizations, and initiatives designed to raise awareness about mental health. Groups like this might set up a table on a school campus common area with pamphlets about mental health or put on activities such as a walk to raise awareness about mental illness. Spaces like this spread a message that people with mental health conditions are treatable and that people affected are like anyone else. Joining initiatives such as these is one way to get involved, meet others who care about mental health, and fight stigma.

Several brave individuals, including some celebrities, have come forward to share their mental health recovery stories to combat the stigma of mental illness. Sharing your story even to someone close to you can also combat stigma.

We can all help to make a change to stigma. Doing things like listening to a friend talk about mental health or not joining in when others poke fun at mental illness can help.

Messages

What messages have you heard about mental health?

_____

_____

_____

How have your views on mental health and mental illness changed since your experiences?

_____

_____

_____

_____

_____

_____

What do you want others to know about mental illness?

_____

_____

_____

_____

_____

_____

Fighting Stigma

Do you want to fight stigma? If so, why?

- ☐ To help others feel less alone
- ☐ To connect with others who care about mental health
- ☐ To feel more comfortable being open about my experiences
- ☐ So that others will feel comfortable reaching out for help

- ☐ _____
- ☐ _____
- ☐ _____

How would you like to fight stigma?

- ☐ Listening to others share their mental health stories
- ☐ Sharing my story
- ☐ Joining a mental health club in the community or at my school
- ☐ Attending a walk or other community event to raise awareness about mental health
- ☐ Giving others good information about mental health
- ☐ Not joking about mental illness
- ☐ Helping others understand why it is not okay to make fun of people who have mental illness
- ☐ Challenging mental health myths

- ☐ _____
- ☐ _____
- ☐ _____

Finding Meaning

A few years ago, a colleague told me about something called "post-traumatic growth." Post-traumatic growth is the positive ways we change and the strengths we sometimes build after a traumatic experience. It does not cancel out the "bad" parts of the experience, but rather gives it meaning.

For some time, I was unsure "why" I had to deal with mental illness. Honestly, I am still unsure why or if there is a why. What I do know, however, is that living with a mental health condition has deepened my compassion for others' suffering. It has given me new outlooks that I otherwise would not have had. Both these gifts have been central to my effectiveness in my career. I have found purpose in helping others living with mental health challenges.

Finding meaning while living with a mental health condition can be complicated. Many of us struggle with symptoms that can overlap with our spirituality. There was a time I feared that God hated me. Still, I found meaning after this and a greater sense of peace in my spirituality.

Making sense of a traumatic event or series of traumatic events is confusing and overwhelming. Mental health conditions are traumatic. Still, many have found meaning after experiencing a mental health crisis.

Meaning can be related to the trauma, such as reflecting on strengthened relationships, a deepened understanding of oneself, or a greater appreciation for life after the trauma. It can also be less clearly connected such as with a spiritual practice, nature, compassion, or following your values.

Some people share that their experience of psychosis has been a spiritual one. This could be a positive experience where someone gains an intensified sense of connection to something greater. It can also be painful. Some see this as a symptom while others have a different view. Whatever your experience has been, know that it is valid.

Spirituality is an expansive idea that reaches through different themes for different people. For some, spirituality is intricately related to religion. For others, it can be found in nature, music, kindness, and other not necessarily religious things. Some people are not religious or spiritual. How you understand your experience and practice (or don't practice) spirituality is totally up to you.

Meaning

· ·

In what ways have you grown since your experience?

- ☐ Better at understanding others' struggles
- ☐ Caring more about people
- ☐ Knowing other people will be there for me
- ☐ Learning a new skill that I otherwise wouldn't have
- ☐ Spiritual growth
- ☐ Greater appreciation for life
- ☐ Building my own strength

☐ _____

☐ _____

☐ _____

In which ways do you practice spirituality?

- ☐ Through attending religious services
- ☐ Through nature
- ☐ Through meditation
- ☐ Through prayer
- ☐ Through compassion
- ☐ Through music
- ☐ Through acts of service to others

☐ _____

☐ _____

☐ _____

In what ways do you hope to continue to grow?

_____

_____

_____

_____

_____

Final Words

Seeking recovery from mental health challenges is like climbing a great mountain. There are times of achievement as well as times of difficulty. Picking up and working through this workbook is a big step on your path to wellness. I appreciate your willingness to take this step and wish you glowing progress on your journey.

Recommended Resources

Memoirs

An Unquiet Mind: A Memoir of Moods and Madness by Dr. Kay Redfield Jamison

The Center Cannot Hold: My Journey Through Madness by Dr. Elyn Sachs

Cracked, Not Broken: Surviving and Thriving After a Suicide Attempt by Kevin Hines

Hearing Voices, Living Fully: Living With the Voices in My Head by Clair Bien

Mind Estranged: My Journey from Schizophrenia and Homelessness to Recovery by Bethany Yeiser

To Cry a Dry Tear: Bill MacPhee's Journey of Hope and Recovery With Schizophrenia by Bill MacPhee

Helplines

Australia

Lifeline Australia: 13 11 14

SANE Helpline: 1800 187 263

Canada

Talk Suicide Canada: 1 833 456 4566

New Zealand

Lifeline: 0800 543 354

UK

Samaritans: 116 123

USA

National Suicide Prevention Lifeline: 988

Organizations and websites
Australia
Early Psychosis Prevention and Intervention Centre: www.oyh.org.au

Emerging Minds: https://emergingminds.com.au

Headspace: https://headspace.org.au

Reachout Australia: www.reachout.org

SANE: www.sane.org

Canada
Canadian Mental Health Association (CMHA): www.cmha.ca

Early Psychosis Intervention: www.earlypsychosis.ca

Mind Your Mind: https://mindyourmind.ca

Schizophrenia Society of Canada (SSC): www.schizophrenia.ca

Stigma-Free Society: www.stigmafreesociety.com

New Zealand
Mental Health Foundation of New Zealand: www.mentalhealth.org.nz

New Zealand Early Intervention Psychosis Society: www.nzeips.co.nz

UK
Early Intervention in Psychosis (EIP) Teams through the NHS: see www.likemind.nhs.uk

Mental Health Foundation: www.mentalhealth.org.uk

SANE: www.sane.org.uk

USA
CureSZ Foundation: www.curesz.org

Mental Health America: www.mhanational.org

National Alliance on Mental Illness: www.nami.org

Schizophrenic.NYC: www.schizophrenic.nyc

Students with Psychosis: www.sws.ngo

Bibliography

Arseneault, L., Cannon, M., Witton, J. and Murray, R.M. (2004) Causal association between cannabis and psychosis: examination of the evidence. *The British Journal of Psychiatry, 184*(2), 110–117.

Beck, A., Grant, P., Inverso, E., Brinen, A.B. and Perivoliotis, D. (2020) *Recovery Oriented Cognitive Therapy for Serious Mental Health Conditions.* New York: The Guilford Press.

Brach, T. (2009) *Radical Compassion: Learning to Love Yourself and Your World with the Practice of RAIN.* New York: Penguin Life.

Copeland, M.E. (1997) *Wellness Recovery Action Plan.* USA: Peach Pr.

Eack, S.M., Greenwald, D.P., Hogarty, S.S., Cooley, S.J., DiBarry, A.L., Montrose, D.M. and Keshavan, M.S. (2009) Cognitive enhancement therapy for early-course schizophrenia: effects of a two-year randomized controlled trial. *Psychiatric Services, 60*(11), 1468–1476.

Gray, L. (2016) *Self-Compassion for Teens: 129 Activities and Practices to Cultivate Kindness.* Eau Claire, WI: PESI Publishing and Media Workbook Edition.

Harper, F.G. (2020) *Unfuck Your Boundaries Workbook: Build Better Relationships through Consent, Communication, and Expressing Your Needs (5-Minute Therapy).* Portland, OR: Microcosm Publishing; Workbook edition.

Ingraham, L.J. and Kety, S.S. (2000) Adoption studies of schizophrenia. *American Journal of Medical Genetics, 97*(1), 18–22.

Kessler, R.C. (2004) The epidemiology of dual diagnosis. *Biological Psychiatry, 56*(10), 730–737.

Kieling, C., Baker-Henningham, H., Belfer, M., Conti, G., Ertem, I., Omigbodun, O., Rohde, L.A., Srinath, S., Ulkuer, N. and Rahman, A. (2011) Child and adolescent mental health worldwide: evidence for action. *The Lancet, 378*(9801), 1515–1525.

Linehan, M.M. (2014) *DBT Skills Training Handouts and Worksheets, Second Edition (2nd ed.).* New York: The Guilford Press.

Luoma, J.B., Hayes, S.C. and Walser, R.D. (2007) *Learning ACT: An Acceptance and Commitment Therapy Skills Training Manual for Therapists.* Oakland, CA: Contextual Press.

Neff, K. (2015) *Self-Compassion: The Proven Power of Being Kind to Yourself.* New York: William Morrow Paperbacks.

Ng, F., Ibrahim, N., Franklin, D., Jordan, G., Lewandowski, F., Fang, F. and Slade, M. (2021) Post-traumatic growth in psychosis: a systematic review and narrative synthesis. *BMC Psychiatry, 21*(1), 1–11.

Petrovsky, N., Ettinger, U., Hill, A., Frenzel, L., Meyhöfer, I., Wagner, M. and Kumari, V. (2014) Sleep deprivation disrupts prepulse inhibition and induces psychosis-like symptoms in healthy humans. *Journal of Neuroscience, 34*(27), 9134–9140.

Pruessner, M., Cullen, A.E., Aas, M. and Walker, E.F. (2017) The neural diathesis-stress model of schizophrenia revisited: An update on recent findings considering illness stage and neurobiological and methodological complexities. *Neuroscience & Biobehavioral Reviews, 73*, 191–218.

Ridgeway, P., McDiremid, D., Davidson, L., Bayes, J. and Ratzlaff, S. (2011) *Pathways to Recovery: A Strengths Recovery Workbook.* Lawrence, KS: University of Kansas, Support Education Group.

Sato, M. (2006) Renaming schizophrenia: a Japanese perspective. *World Psychiatry, 5*(1), 53.

Slade, M. and Longden, E. (2015) Empirical evidence about recovery and mental health. *BMC Psychiatry, 15*(1), 1–14.

Wright, N., Turkington, D., Kelly, O., Davies, D., Jacobs, A. and Hopton, J. (2014) *Treating Psychosis.* New York: New Harbinger Publications.